# Type 2 Diabetes Instant Pot Cookbook

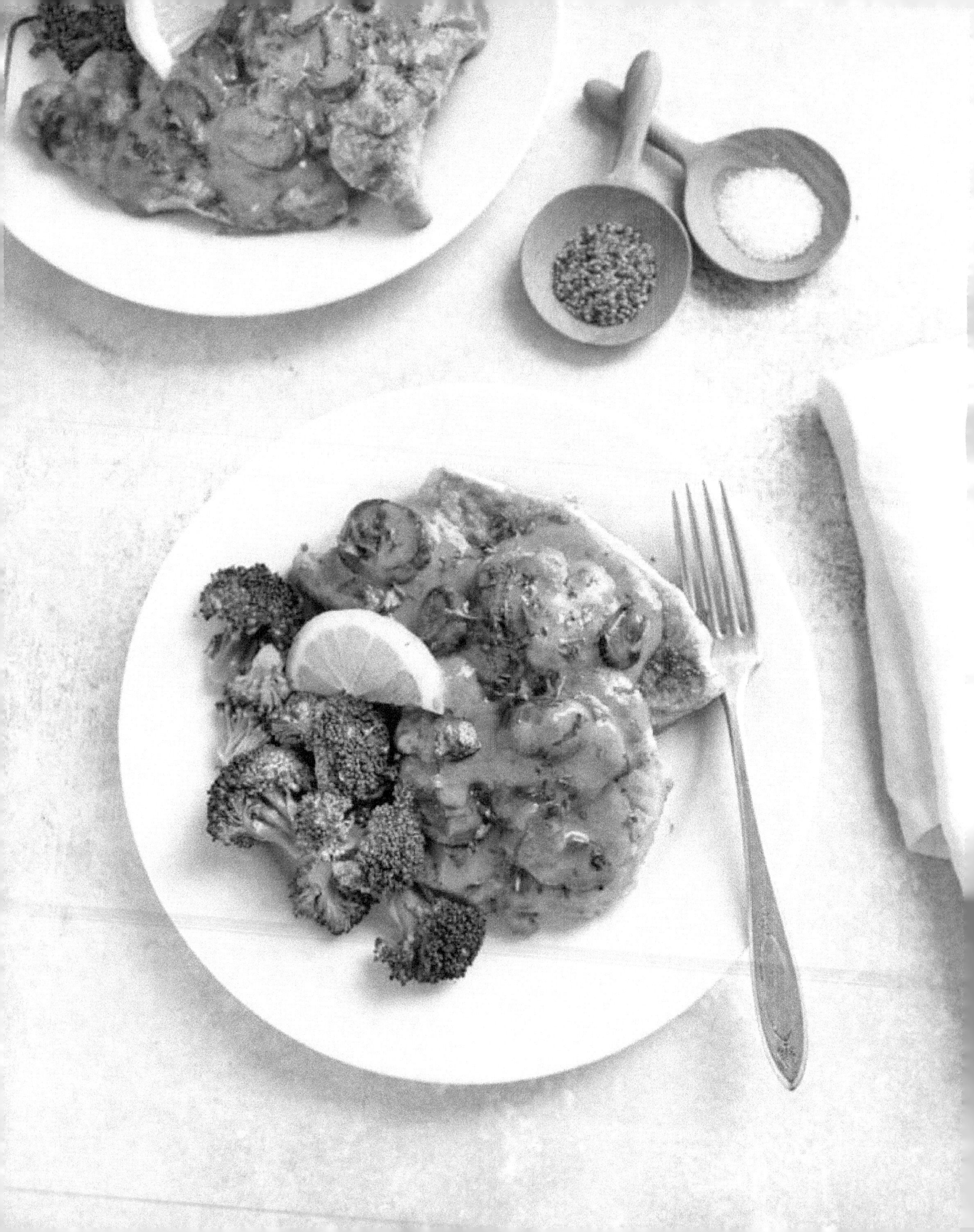

# Type 2 Diabetes Instant Pot Cookbook

## Quick and Easy Instant Pot Pressure Cooker Recipes to Lower Blood Pressure and Manage Type 2 Diabetes

Ronald Tuck

# CONTENT


**Introduction   1**

**Chapter 1   Diabetes 101   2**

**Chapter 2   The Instant Pot for Diabetes   10**

**Chapter 3   Breakfast   14**

**Chapter 4   Snacks and Appetizers   30**

**Chapter 5   Soups and Stews   39**

**Chapter 6   Vegetables and Sides   55**

**Chapter 7   Meatless Mains   63**

**Chapter 8   Poultry   78**

**Chapter 9   Meat   90**

**Chapter 10   Fish and Seafood   102**

**Chapter 11   Desserts   109**

**Chapter 12   Staples   116**

**Appendix 1   Measurement Conversion Chart   123**

**Appendix 2   Instant Pot Cooking Timetable   124**

**Appendix 3   The Dirty Dozen and Clean Fifteen   126**


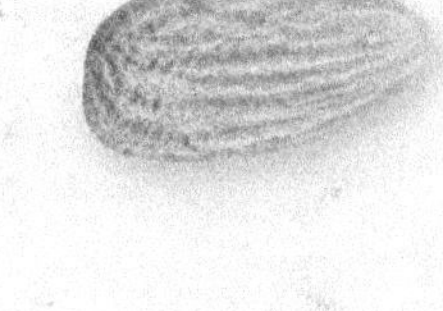
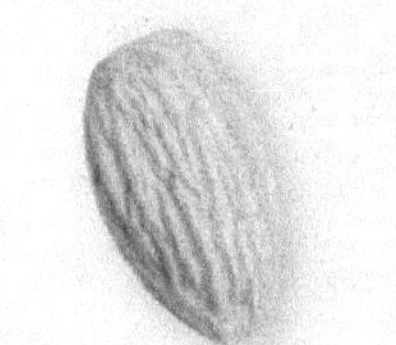
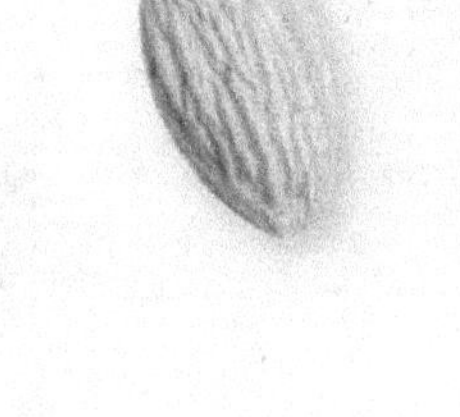
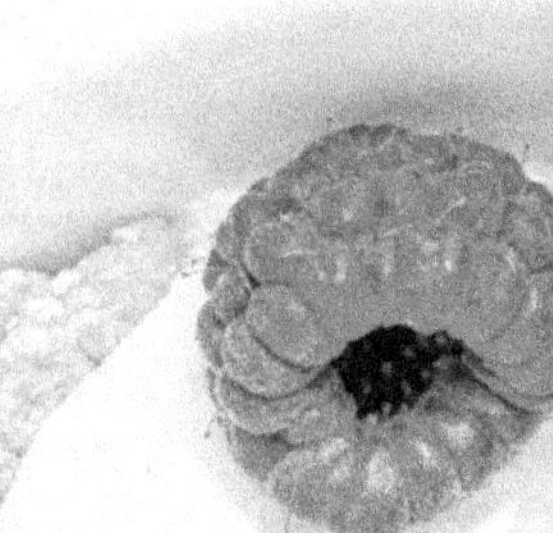
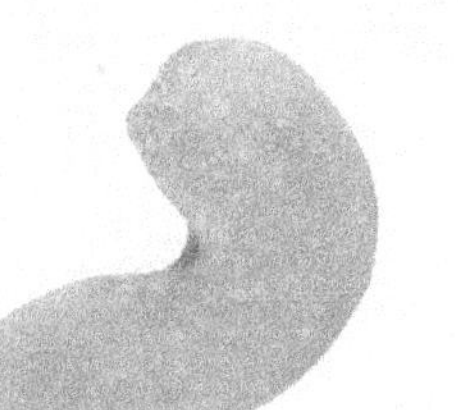
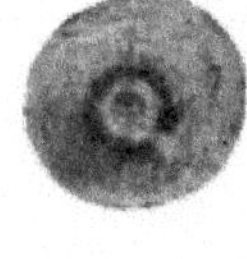
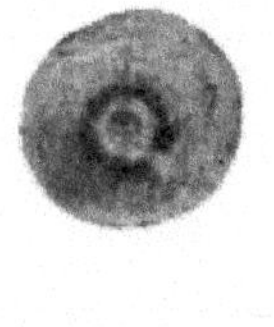
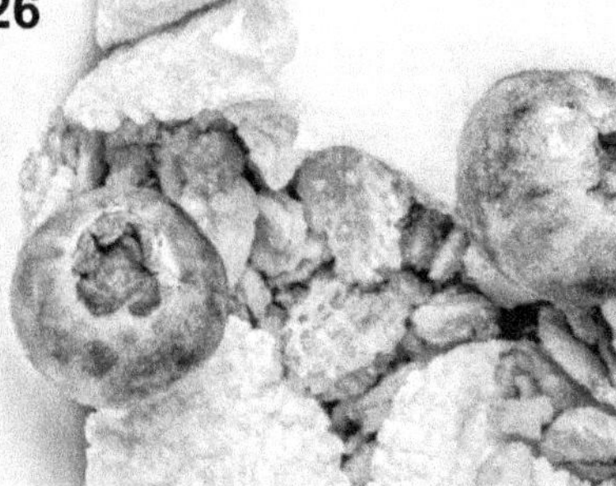
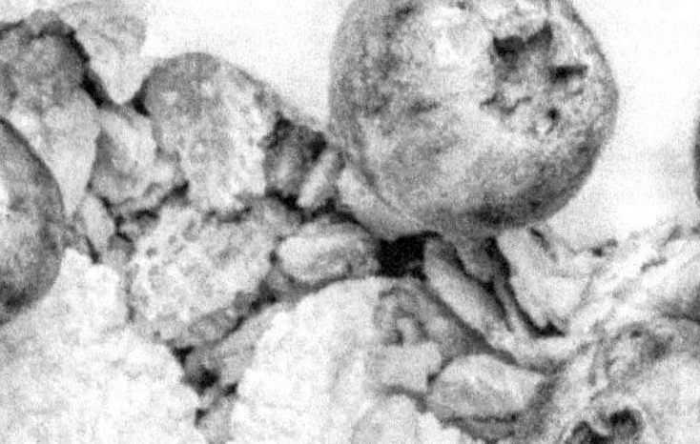

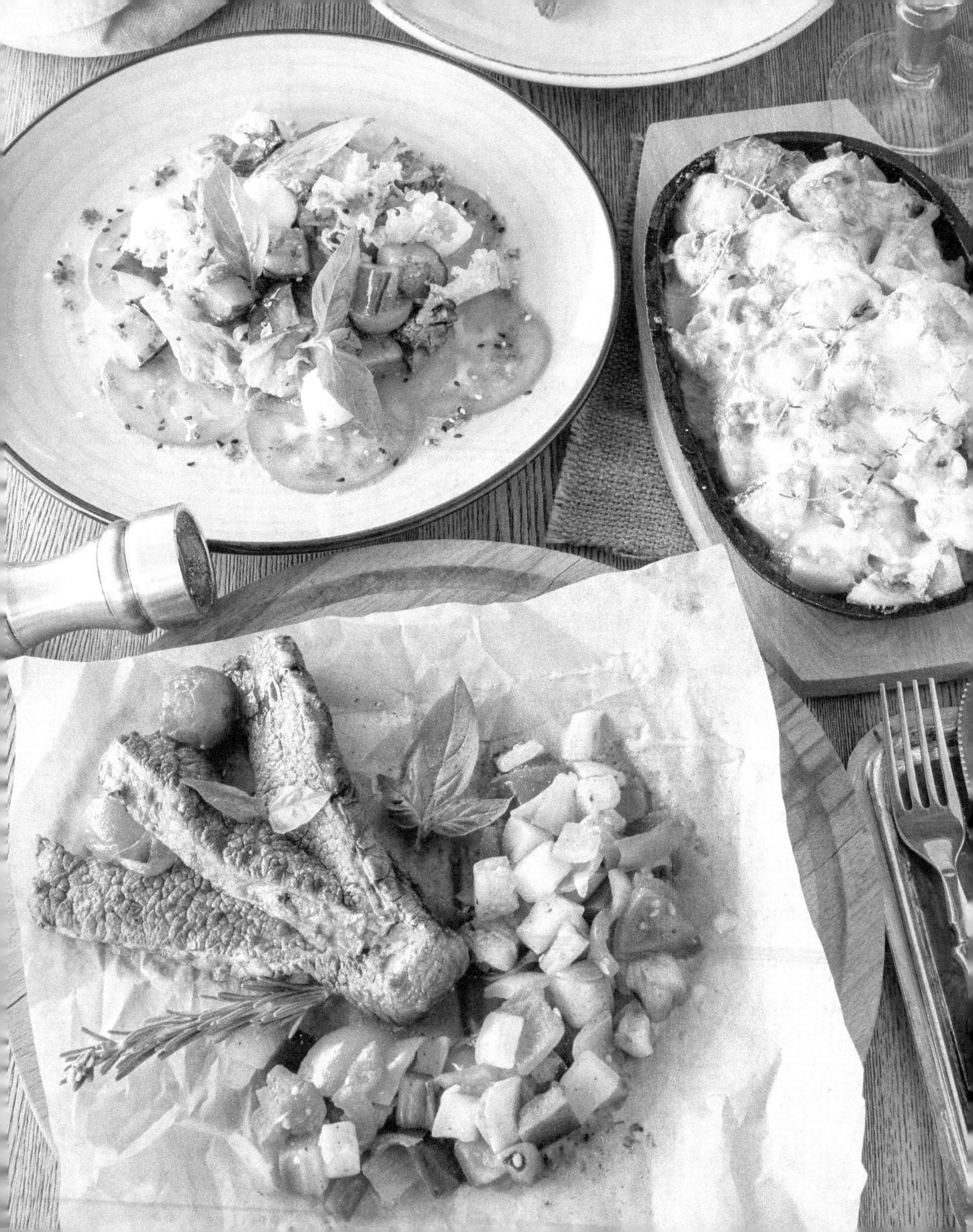

# Introduction

Have you just been diagnosed with diabetes, or have you been living with this diagnosis for a long time? Either way, you're probably looking for some interesting ways to improve the foods you eat while sticking to a healthy diabetic diet. If this sounds like you, then you're in good company!

Many individuals who are diagnosed with diabetes worry that they won't be able to eat anything delicious anymore. But don't worry—this simply isn't true! Just because you're living with diabetes, that doesn't mean you have to eat boring, bland foods for the rest of your life.

It also doesn't mean you have to concoct elaborate meals every time you cook, either. With the help of your Instant Pot, you can manage your diabetes diagnosis while keeping your meals and snacks quick and easy at the same time.

In this book, you'll find information about diabetic meal planning and nutrition as well as some basics to help you get started with your Instant Pot. From there, you'll discover tons of delicious, helpful, and easy recipes you can make with your Instant Pot that will fit well into just about any diabetic diet plan.

Read on to find out more and get started cooking!

# Chapter 1 Diabetes 101

In this chapter, we'll take a brief look at diabetes and help you better understand your diagnosis. Be sure to check out the sections on diabetic dieting and which foods to eat and avoid later on in this chapter as well.

## What Does It Mean to Be Diagnosed with Diabetes?

If you've been diagnosed with diabetes, chances are good you already have some basic understanding of what this disease means. But many adults with a diabetes diagnosis are unclear about the meaning or find themselves with more questions than answers moving forward. If this sounds like you, then don't worry—you're not alone.

Diabetes is a disease that Is related to the content of sugar in your blood, which is also called blood glucose. Although blood glucose is an important part of the energy your body receives from food and uses every day, it's very easy for blood glucose levels to run too high. This happens when your body doesn't produce enough insulin to help convert the sugar in food to energy for your body.

In other words, when your body is unable to use glucose for energy, it stays in your blood and causes your blood sugar to rise. This can become very dangerous if left unchecked, and permanent high levels of blood glucose in your body can cause you to become diabetic.

There are two main types of diabetes. Type 1 diabetes occurs from birth or from a very young age, while type 2 diabetes can occur at any point and is more common in older adults. Both types require multiple methods of treatment for the individual to stay alive and well.

## Treatments for Diabetes

These are just some of the treatments you may incorporate as you work toward managing your diabetes.

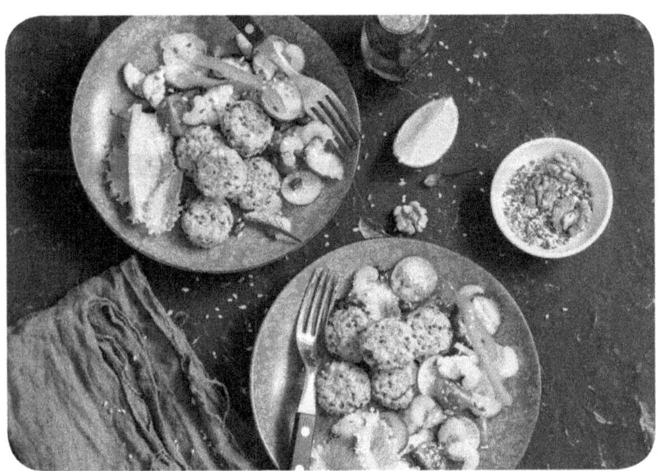

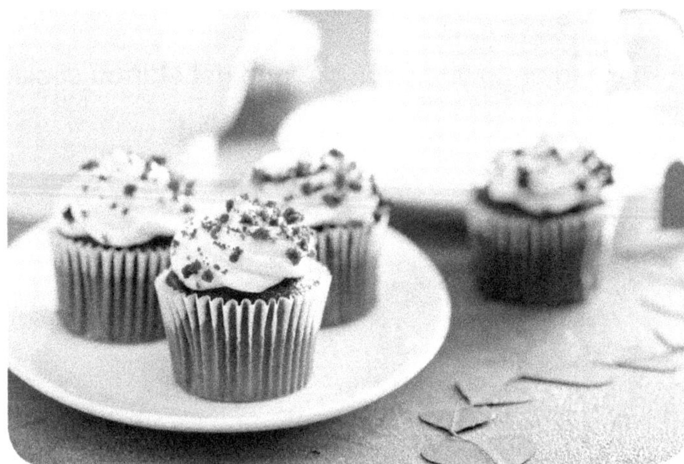

## Medical Treatment

Anyone with type 1 or type 2 diabetes should monitor their blood sugar levels and work with a trusted doctor to figure out the right medical treatment plan. You will also need to have your A1C levels checked via lab work frequently.

In addition to blood sugar checks, you may need to go on insulin injections if your diabetes is severe. Type 1 diabetics will probably need to stay on insulin from initial diagnosis and throughout the rest of their lives. Type 2 diabetics may be able to avoid insulin through other treatment options.

## Diet Treatment

There are many methods of managing your diet, and watching what you eat can play a major role in helping you treat and take care of your diabetes. When you stick to a carefully planned diet that is high in nutritional value, you can improve your diabetes symptoms and feel better at the same time.

It's important to eat plenty of vegetables and some fruits on a diabetes diet. You should also focus on whole grains and leaner proteins, while avoiding proteins that are known for a higher fat count. Carbohydrates and sugars should be cut down significantly, but still eaten in moderation, while high-fiber foods with lots of nutritional value should make up the bulk of your diet.

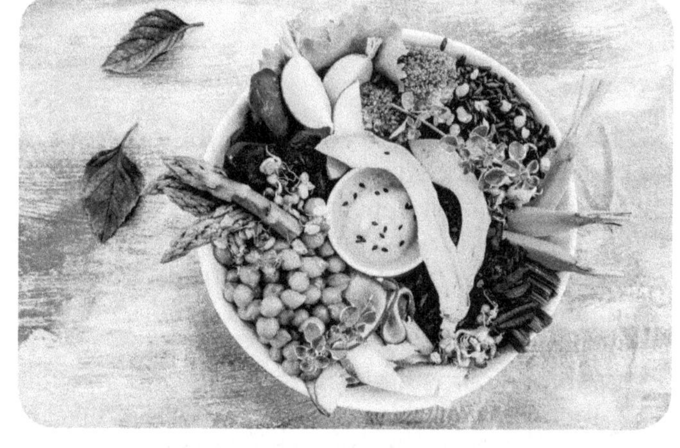

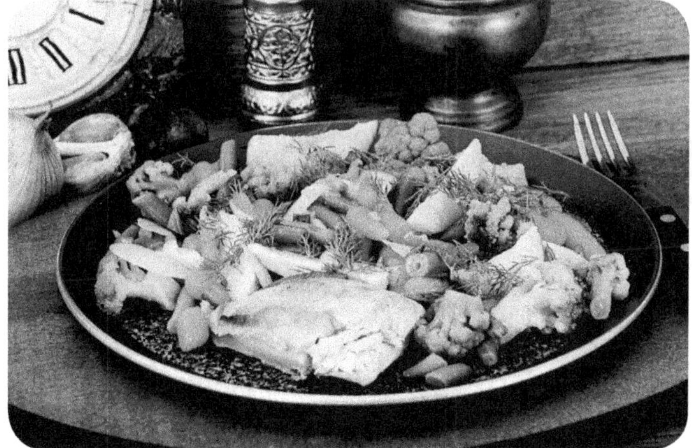

Understanding what to eat when you're diabetic can be extremely challenging, especially at first. This is why it's a good idea to formulate the perfect meal plan from day one by putting together an arsenal of go-to recipes. This way, you'll never find yourself without the right food for any given day or meal, and you can always have a recipe ready for just about any situation that comes your way.

Along with monitoring your diet, you should also add exercise and physical activity to your diabetes treatment plan. When you exercise, your body utilizes the sugar from food by turning it into energy to power your activity. By doing this regularly, you can cut down on the amount of blood glucose in your body and reduce the effects of your diabetes.

Your doctor can help you figure out the best exercise plan based on your current activity levels and your other health concerns. Most individuals with diabetes should try to exercise at least 15 minutes per day, but some may need more activity than this.

## Diabetes Nutrients

Pay attention to these nutrients, as they are all some of the most important in a diabetic diet.

**Macros**

**Carbohydrates:** Carbs can give you energy. They help your body maintain its metabolism and improve brain functionality at the same time. There are two different types of carbs, however, and it's important to focus on the "healthy carbs" when you're eating a diabetic diet.

- Fibrous carbs are slow to digest and are much healthier for you than the alternative. On a diabetic diet, you should focus as much as possible on fibrous carbs to cut down on the feeling of hunger throughout the day and improve your physical health and energy.
- Starchy carbs come from starches and sugars, and they are not very healthy. They can give you a quick energy boost and may be necessary at some points in the day depending on how much you exercise, but they shouldn't make up the bulk of your diet.

**Proteins:** Proteins are extremely important in ensuring your body has enough energy to get through the day. If you're exercising regularly, you need to eat enough protein to help your muscle rebuild after you work out, too.

- Choose healthy sources of protein that come from lean animal meats whenever possible. Poultry, fish, and eggs are good options.
- You can also get protein from some plants, such as mushrooms or broccoli.

**Fat:** It's easy to think that all fats should be avoided, but this simply isn't the case. Fat is a nutrient, just like all the others on this list, and you shouldn't cut it out of your diet altogether. You should, however, try to choose healthy sources of fat whenever possible.

- Lean fat sources are best. It's ideal to stick to fish and eggs as well as plant sources of fats (such as avocado) whenever possible.
- Animal fats may be too rich for a diabetic diet. However, some leaner sources of animal fats, such as poultry, can be useful.

**Sodium:** Eating too much sodium can cause high blood pressure in diabetics (and in non-diabetics as well). However, your body needs some sodium in order to function properly.

**Potassium:** Potassium is one of the nutrients your body requires in order to produce insulin. When your potassium is too low, you will feel the effects of your diabetes more fully. Eating enough potassium from healthy plant sources is a great way to improve your overall wellbeing when you are diabetic.

**Magnesium:** When your body is resistant to insulin, it may also have low magnesium levels. You should focus on foods that are high in magnesium to keep yourself as well as possible.

**Calcium:** Calcium comes from milk, eggs, and several plant sources. You need plenty of calcium in your diet every day, so be sure to stock up on these healthy foods.

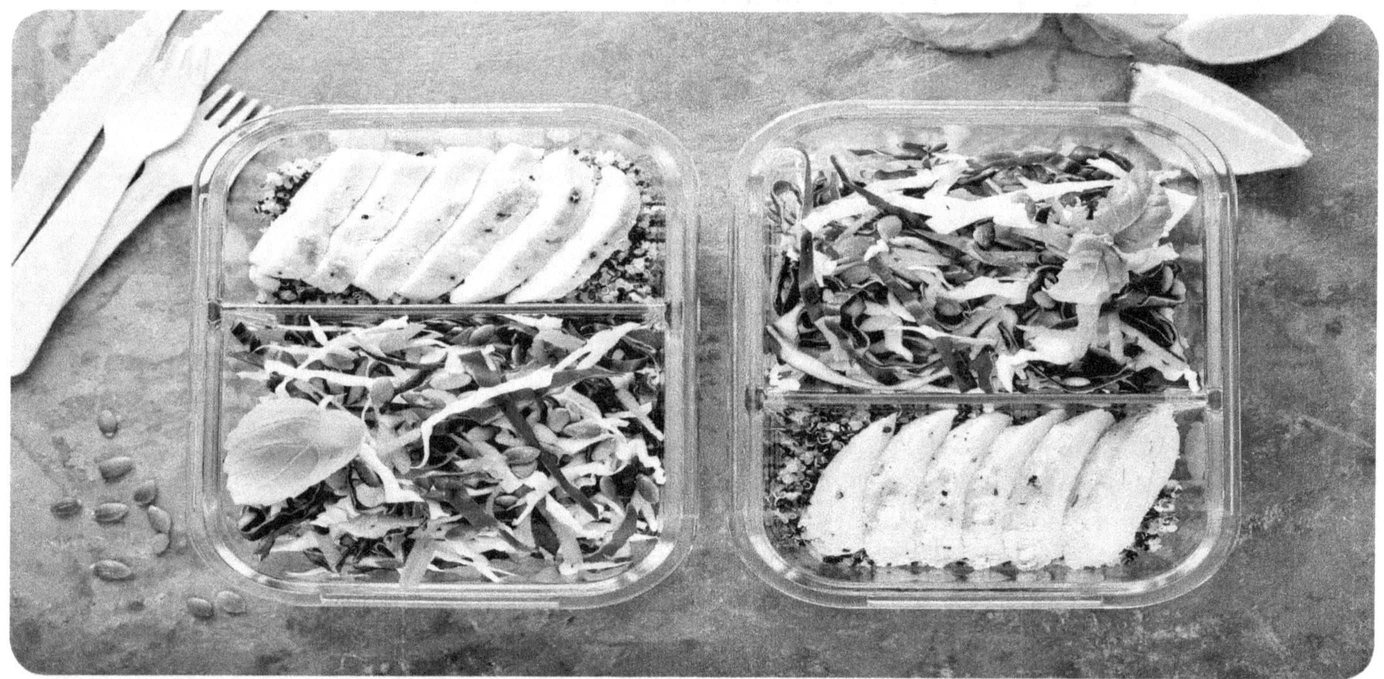

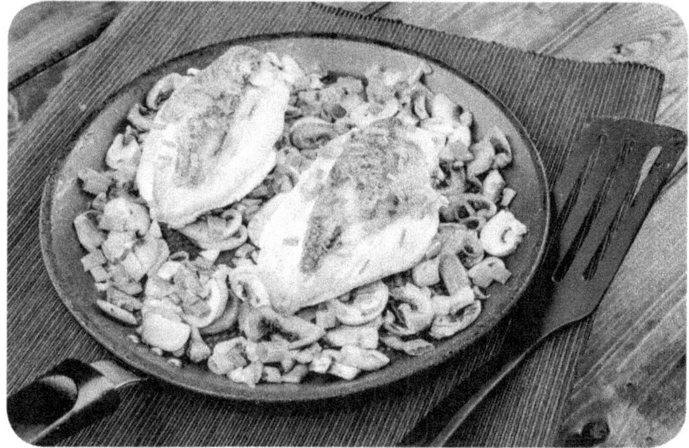

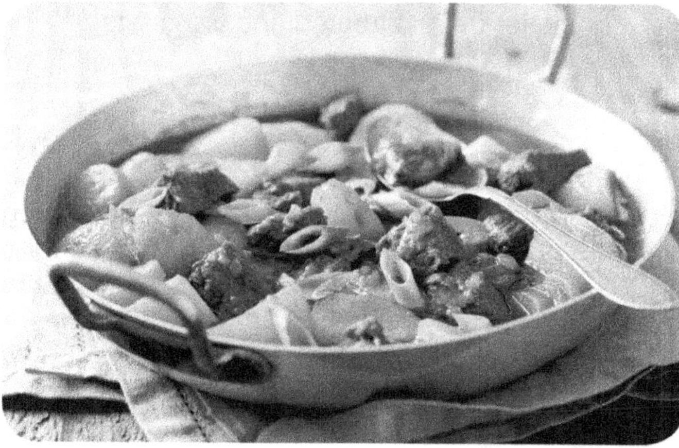

## Carb Counting

- Carb counting is one of the most common methods of managing diabetes through your diet. To carb count, you should check the number of carbohydrate grams in every food you eat and then match your insulin dosage to that number.
- Individuals who use an insulin pump should use an insulin-to-carb ratio to determine their dosage after every meal.
- Those who are not on insulin but still want to count carbs to help manage their diabetes can do so by using carbohydrate choices instead. Each choice should account for roughly 15 grams of carbohydrates, and sticking to this plan can help you manage your diabetes and prevent the need for insulin injections too.
- Others use the plate method to make sure they aren't eating too many carbs at a given meal. To do this, make sure the foods you eat that contain carbs make up no more than one quarter of your plate.
- The number of carbs you need in a meal or in a day will depend on your individual diabetes diagnosis, your age, your weight, and any other health conditions you may be dealing with at the same time. For this reason, it's necessary to work with a medical professional to make sure you're eating the right amount of carbs and other nutrients every day.

## How to Read Labels

- Learning how to read labels is crucial in managing your diabetes through your diet. Check the labels first for ingredients that are known for being good for your heart, and learn how to recognize fats and oils that are unhealthy.
- Check for sugar content, but don't forget to check for carbohydrate content as well. Carbohydrates include natural sugar, complex carbs, and fiber, all of which are important to consider in your diabetic diet.
- Remember that sugar-free doesn't necessarily mean healthy. Some sugar-free foods are still very high in carbs, calories, or fat content.
- Fat-free isn't always healthy either. Check labels to find monounsaturated and polyunsaturated fats, which are healthier than saturated and trans fats.

**Nutrition Facts**

8 servings per container

**Serving size    2/3 cup (55g)**

Amount per serving

**Calories    230**

| | % Daily Value* |
|---|---|
| **Total Fat** 8g | 10% |
| Saturated Fat 1g | 5% |
| *Trans* Fat 0g | |
| **Cholesterol** 0mg | 0% |
| **Sodium** 160mg | 7% |
| **Total Carbohydrate** 37g | 13% |
| Dietary Fiber 4g | 14% |
| Total Sugars 12g | |
| Includes 10g Added Sugars | 20% |
| **Protein** 3g | |
| Vitamin D 2mcg | 10% |
| Calcium 260mg | 20% |
| Iron 8mg | 45% |
| Potassium 240mg | 6% |

* The % Daily Value (DV) tells you how much a nutrient in a serving of food contributes to a daily diet. 2,000 calories a day is used for general nutrition advice.

## Foods to Eat

This list does not contain every food you can eat on a diabetic diet, but it can help you get started understand what to focus on when meal planning.

- Berries and citrus. Berries are very good for you because they contain lots of antioxidants. They also include vitamin C, potassium, and manganese, and some also contain vitamin K. Citrus also contains antioxidants and lots of vitamin C as well as plenty of potassium.
- Beans. Beans are packed with protein and are great at reducing hunger. They are a healthy starch that also include complex carbs, which are better for you than other types of carbs. Beans can also help you regulate your cholesterol and get enough magnesium in your diet. Just be sure

to prepare beans that do not have salt added.
- Whole grains. Instead of refined or processed grains, stick with whole grains. They are high in fiber content and contain healthy carbohydrates. Additionally, since they take longer for your body to digest, they help balance your blood glucose levels over time.
- Leafy greens. You should eat some leafy greens every day whenever possible. They are very healthy and contain tons of nutrients, including calcium, potassium, vitamin A, and other vitamins. Leafy greens also contain antioxidants and are helpful in regulating your digestive system at the same time as they improve your blood glucose levels.
- Fatty fish. Pack your diet with protein sourced from fatty fish whenever possible. Fatty fish contains omega-3 fatty acids, which are important for your brain and heart. They also contain healthy fats.
- Sweet potatoes. Sweet potatoes have healthy fiber as well as vitamin C, vitamin A, and lots of potassium. They don't increase your blood sugar like starchy white potatoes do, and they can be prepared in a lot of different tasty methods to keep them interesting as well.

## Foods to Avoid

Below, you'll find some of the most common foods you should avoid when you are diabetic.
- Foods that are very high in carbs. You do need enough carbs every day to help balance your blood sugar, but high carbs can throw off your blood glucose more than help it. Work to make sure you're managing your carbs appropriately.
- Saturated and trans fats. These are usually found in fried, baked, and oily foods like French fries or donuts. They are "bad fats" and should be avoided.
- Drinks with sugar or with sugar substitutes. Soda, energy drinks, sweet tea, or very sugary coffee drinks should be avoided.
- Overly salty food. Too much salt (or sodium) in your food can cause your blood pressure to rise to dangerously high levels. Everyone, diabetic or not, should aim for 2300mg of sodium per day or, ideally, less.
- Processed sugar. Sometimes also called refined sugar, this ingredient is usually found in desserts. It is not the same as sugar found in milk or fruit.
- Alcohol in larger quantities. It's usually okay to have one drink with a meal, but too much alcohol should be avoided as well.
- Processed or refined grains. Just like refined sugar, refined grain can contain too much sugar or carb content and negatively affect your blood glucose.
- Certain plant starches and sugars. Potatoes, melons, pineapple, and pumpkin all contain more starch and sugar than is healthy for a diabetic diet, except in extreme moderation.

## Watching What You Eat

This section can help you better understand how to watch what you eat and which foods to pay extra attention to when planning your meals for the week.

## Portion Control

- Portion control is by far the most important method of controlling your diabetes symptoms through your diet. By watching your portions, you can improve your overall health and wellbeing, sometimes without the use of medication at all.
- Always read labels to make sure you're eating the proper serving size of any food or ingredient.
- Invest in a food scale and use it to weigh proper portions. Eyeballing your portion sizes can quickly lead to overdoing it.
- Use smaller plates to help yourself feel like you're getting larger portions. This can also help you manage your portions by simply not loading up a larger plate with a lot of extra food.
- Be careful when going out to eat, especially at buffets. Consider asking for a to-go bag before you ever start eating, so you can make sure to save some for later.

## Alcohol

- Alcohol contains sugars, carbs, and calories, all of which may factor into your diabetic diet. Since liquid carbs are absorbed fast, they don't really make a difference in balancing your blood sugar, but the calories present in alcohol still add up.
- Many medications used to treat diabetes interact badly with alcohol. Drinking alcohol with these medications can lead to low blood sugar, which can be very dangerous.
- It's usually okay to have one drink with a meal when you are diabetic. However, multiple drinks in a day, or drinks on an empty stomach, should be avoided.

## Sugar Substitutes

- It can be tempting to use sugar substitutes as part of your diabetic diet. However, most of the time, it's better to skip these unless you're sure you can choose one of the healthier options. Some sugar substitutes can actually increase your risk of worsening your diabetes, especially when consumed for a long time.
- Some of the healthiest sugar substitutes available are stevia, monk fruit, coconut palm sugar, and date sugar. These all come from natural sources and some even contain antioxidants that can help you stay healthier.
- Stevia increases your body's insulin production and improves your blood sugar levels.
- Monk fruit is a sweetener made from pressed or extracted monk fruit, making it a good, natural way to sweeten your food.
- Coconut palm sugar and date sugar are made of dried and ground natural ingredients. Date sugar is also a good source of fiber.
- Sugar alcohols are types of sweeteners that can be found naturally in some plants, although most are made from chemicals. These include xylitol, sorbitol, and sucralose, among others. Sweeteners like Sweet-N-Low or Splenda contain these sugar alcohols.
- Although sugar alcohols are synthetic, they are actually better for you than some other artificial sweeteners. Your body can metabolize them without the use of insulin, and they can also be partially digested. Both of these factors cut down on risks associated with using sugar alcohols as sweeteners.
- Of the sugar substitutes on the market, stevia is the healthiest option for most diabetic individuals.

For now, we'll leave this chapter with some important tips that can help you manage your diabetes diagnosis. These tips are necessary to keep in mind when working toward a healthier method of living with your diagnosis.

- Always work with a trusted doctor, and consider working with a nutritionist as well. Medical professionals can give you the best advice about your specific needs.
- Eat well-balanced meals and don't be afraid to choose healthy snacks if you get hungry in between meals.
- Always plan your meals ahead of time.
- Go grocery shopping with a list to avoid purchasing unhealthy snack foods.
- Get enough exercise for your age, weight, and other health conditions.
- Hydrate, hydrate, hydrate! Drink plenty of water every day.
- If you are on insulin or other medication, always take it as directed by your doctor, and make sure you have extra doses with you at all times.

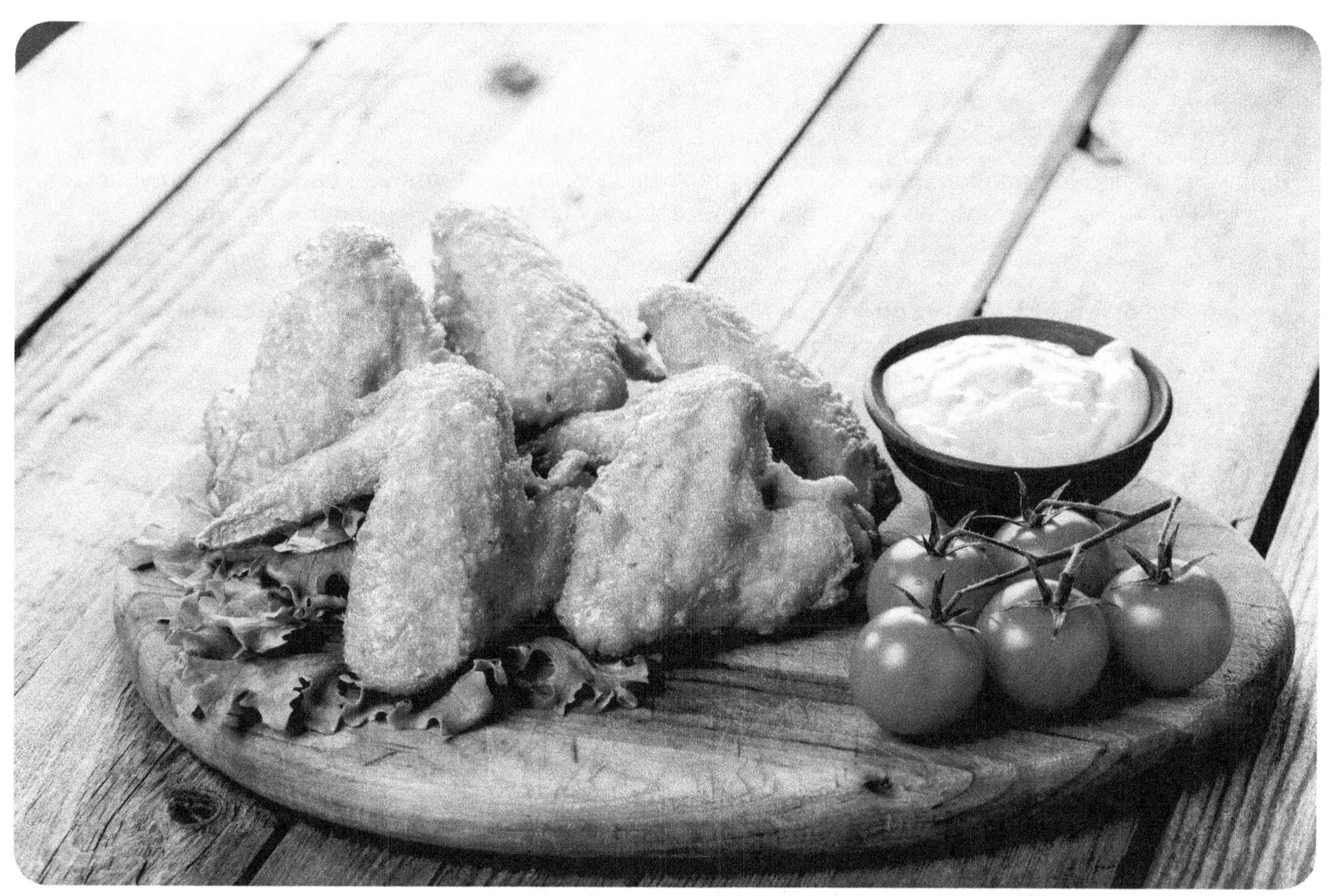

Now that you've had a chance to brush up on the basics when it comes to diabetes and your diet, it's time to learn a little bit more about the Instant Pot. This unique and innovative cooking appliance can help you create the perfect diabetic meals and snacks all in one convenient place. Check out this chapter to find out more.

## Why Instant Pot Cooking?

If you've never tried cooking with an Instant Pot before, you might find yourself wondering whether or not it's really worth it. However, most people who use an Instant Pot regularly are more than happy with the results and enjoy the ease with which they can prepare a variety of foods.

When you cook with an Instant Pot, you can save time and make your favorite meals more easily than ever before. Instant Pots also don't take up much room, so you don't have to worry about a large appliance on your countertops either. There are tons of reasons to try Instant Pot cooking, and if you're getting started with a diabetic diet, you may find even more benefits than you expect!

## Buttons and Features

Below, you'll find information on some of the many buttons and features you can enjoy with your Instant Pot. Although all models are slightly different, they share many similarities as well.

- **Instant Pot models all have buttons that allow you to choose the type of food you're cooking or the type of cooking you want to perform. These may vary slightly depending on the model of Instant Pot you have, but they usually include:**

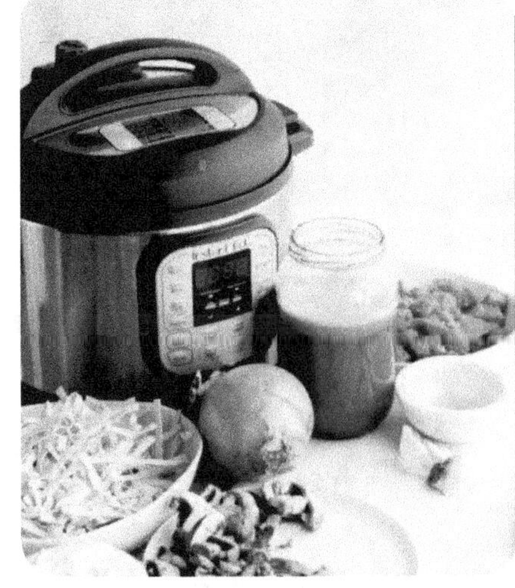

- **Manual**
- **Sauté**
- **Slow Cook**
- **Poultry**
- **Bean/Chili**
- **Meat/Stew**
- **Soup**
- **Rice**
- **Multigrain**
- **Porridge**
- **Steam**
- **Yogurt**
- **Instant Pots also have buttons that let you control the pressure level and amount of time you'll need to cook the food in question.**
- **Some Instant Pots have digital displays and others do not, but they all have user-friendly button controls on the front of the pot that make them easy to understand.**

- **Instant Pots also come with a sealing lid that has a steam release button. The auto-sealing lid ensures the perfect, safe seal for every pressure-cooking task, and the steam release vents steam safely away from any users.**
- **Your Instant Pot will also come with a stainless-steel cooking pot that is easy to clean and take care of.**

## Benefits of Instant Pot Recipes for Diabetes

The Instant Pot is convenient for any home chef, but for a diabetic diet, it has even more uses.

- Easy, quick meal prep. The Instant Pot makes it easy for you to create delicious meals without much time. Since the cooking pot is insulated, it heats up fast, and it can boil and cook more quickly than other cooking appliances.
- Lots of options. With so many different buttons and modes to choose from, your Instant Pot can help you find unique and tasty ways to enjoy the foods that are healthy for your diabetic diet. You'll be able to prepare tons of meals all with just one pot.
- Nutrient retention. Since the food in a pressure cooker like the Instant Pot cooks fast, it retains a lot more of its nutrients and vitamins than food prepared in other methods. This is great for diabetic dieting, since it means you'll be able to get all the healthy ingredients you need to safely and effectively manage your diabetes through the food you eat.
- Plenty of flavor. Best of all, when you cook with an Instant Pot, this cooking method also retains a lot of flavors. Your food doesn't have to be boring or dull, and you don't have to be stuck with the same few bland meals just because you're eating a diabetes-friendly diet. Your Instant Pot can help your food become more flavorful and vibrant than ever before!

## Maintenance

Proper maintenance for your Instant Pot is important in ensuring it remains functional and healthy for you to cook with. However, maintenance is quick and easy when you take care of your Instant Pot. The lid, steaming rack, sealing ring, and cooking pot portion of the Instant Pot are all dishwasher safe. You can also wash them by hand with hot, soapy water if you prefer (or if you don't have a dishwasher).

Before cleaning any parts of your Instant Pot, make sure to unplug it and let it cool fully for your safety. After cleaning, be sure everything is completely dry before replacing it.

Do not use scrubbing pads on the inner cooking pot. Soak it in water or white vinegar if you're having trouble removing some stains from the pot.

Remove the silicone cap from the float valve before rinsing it out. Replace the float valve before operating the Instant Pot again.

Always make sure your sealing ring is properly reinstalled after cleaning to prevent any accidents with the Instant Pot. Replace it every year or sooner if it becomes cracked or damaged.

Wipe down the outside base of the Instant Pot with a damp cloth. Never submerge the base in water and never use a soaking cloth on it.

Instant Pot Tips and Warnings

Keep these important warnings and tips in mind to ensure the safe operation of your Instant Pot.

- **Always thoroughly read the instruction manual before you start using the Instant Pot.**

- Do not fill the Instant Pot all the way to the max fill line, especially if you're using it to cook pasta, oats, or rice.
- Take care to never open the Instant Pot in your face or in the direction of anyone else either.
- Never cook with less than one cup of liquid in the Instant Pot.
- Never leave home with your Instant Pot running. You don't have to stand there and watch it the whole time it cooks, but you should be available in case anything goes wrong.
- Like any type of pressure cooker, the Instant Pot can potentially explode when misused. Be sure you understand all of its safety features to prevent this from happening.
- If you use the quick release function on your Instant Pot, be sure to wear a protective glove so you can avoid steam burns on your hands.

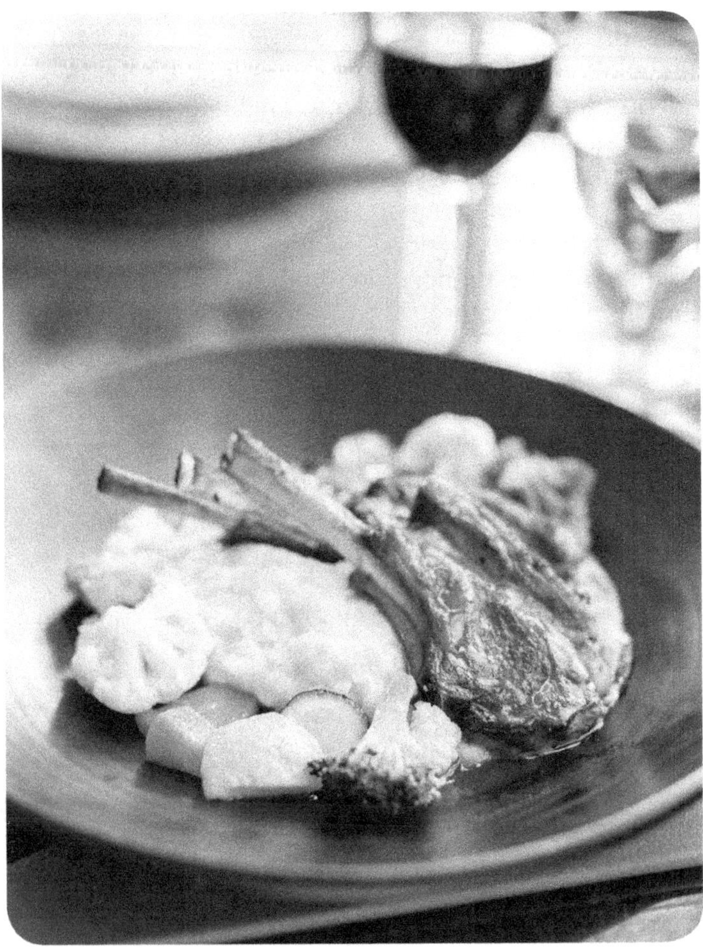

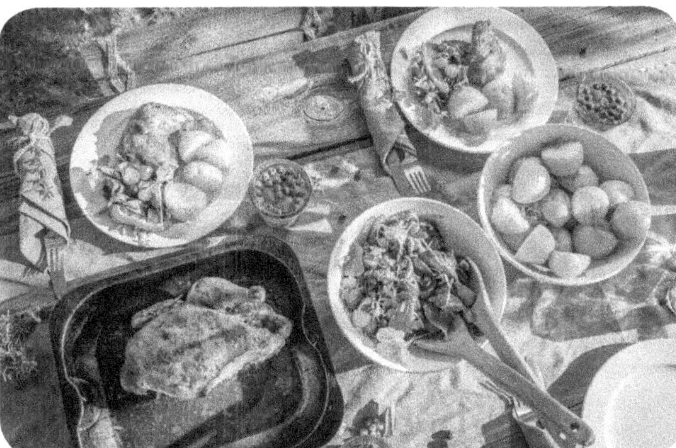

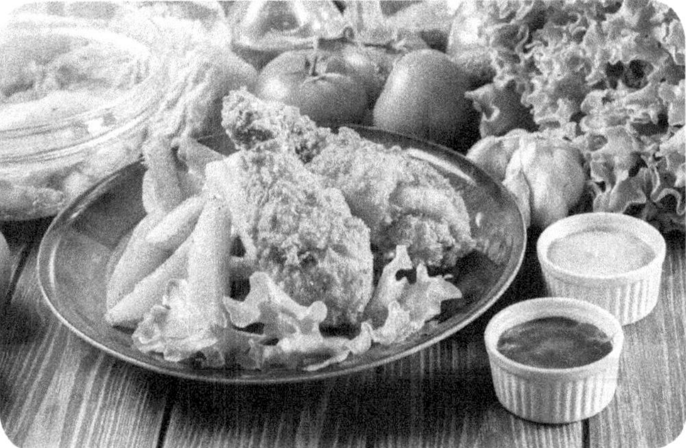

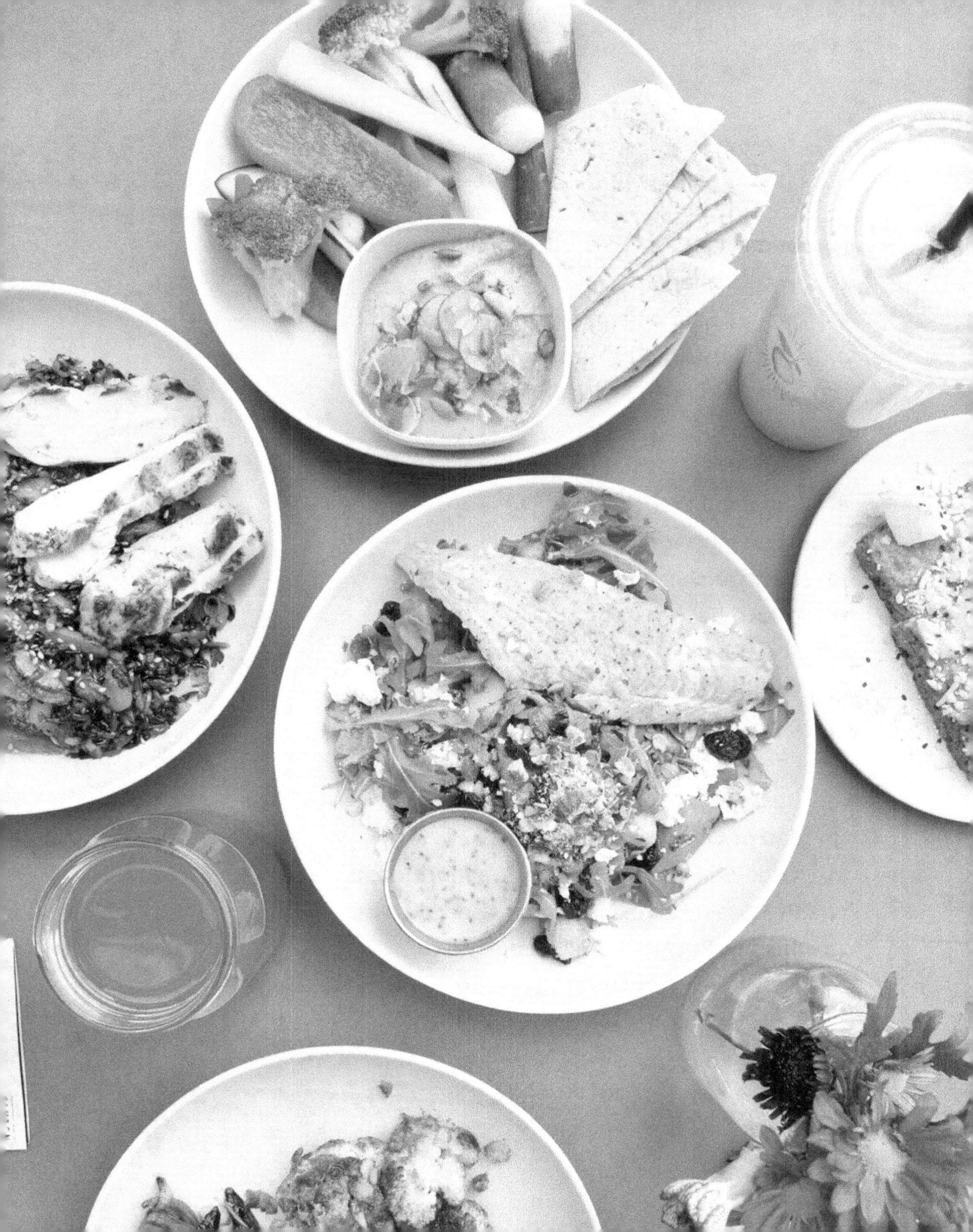

# Chapter 3 Breakfast

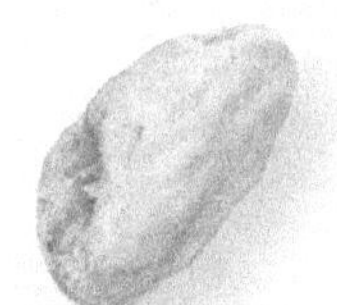

1   Gouda Egg Casserole with Canadian Bacon   15

2   Cynthia's Yogurt   15

3   Smoked Salmon and Asparagus Quiche Cups   16

4   Southwestern Egg Casserole   16

5   Shakshuka with Swiss Chard   17

6   Tropical Steel Cut Oats   17

7   Blueberry Oat Mini Muffins   18

8   Cinnamon French Toast   18

9   Baked Eggs   19

10   Easy Quiche   19

11   Potato-Bacon Gratin   20

12   Shredded Potato Omelet   20

13   Coddled Huevos Rancheros   21

14   Cranberry Almond Grits   21

15   Egg Bites with Sausage and Peppers   22

16   Best Steel-Cut Oats   23

17   Carrot Cake Oatmeal   23

18   Coddled Eggs and Smoked Salmon Toasts   24

19   Breakfast Farro with Berries and Walnuts   24

20   Instant Pot Hard-Boiled Eggs   25

21   Free Apple Cinnamon Cake   25

22   Breakfast Millet with Nuts and Strawberries   26

23   Poached Eggs   26

24   Greek Frittata with Peppers, Kale, and Feta   27

# Gouda Egg Casserole with Canadian Bacon

**Prep time: 12 minutes | Cook time: 20 minutes | Serves 4**

Nonstick cooking spray
½ cup shredded smoked Gouda cheese
6 large eggs
¼ teaspoon kosher salt
¼ teaspoon dry mustard

1 slice whole grain bread, toasted
3 slices Canadian bacon, chopped
¼ cup half-and-half
¼ teaspoon freshly ground black pepper

1. Spray a 6-inch cake pan with cooking spray, or if the pan is nonstick, skip this step. If you don't have a 6-inch cake pan, any bowl or pan that fits inside your pressure cooker should work.
2. Crumble the toast into the bottom of the pan. Sprinkle with the cheese and Canadian bacon.
3. In a medium bowl, whisk together the eggs, half-and-half, salt, pepper, and dry mustard.
4. Pour the egg mixture into the pan. Loosely cover the pan with aluminum foil.
5. Pour 1½ cups water into the electric pressure cooker and insert a wire rack or trivet. Place the covered pan on top of the rack.
6. Close and lock the lid of the pressure cooker. Set the valve to sealing.
7. Cook on high pressure for 20 minutes.
8. When the cooking is complete, hit Cancel and quick release the pressure.
9. Once the pin drops, unlock and remove the lid.
10. Carefully transfer the pan from the pressure cooker to a cooling rack and let it sit for 5 minutes.
11. Cut into 4 wedges and serve.

**Per Serving**

calories: 247 | fat: 15g | protein: 20g | carbs: 8g | sugars: 1g | fiber: 1g | sodium: 717mg

# Cynthia's Yogurt

**Prep time: 10 minutes | Cook time: 8 hours | Serves 16**

1 gallon low-fat milk

¼ cup low-fat plain yogurt with active cultures

1. Pour milk into the inner pot of the Instant Pot.
2. Lock lid, move vent to sealing, and press the yogurt button. Press Adjust till it reads "boil".
3. When boil cycle is complete (about 1 hour), check the temperature. It should be at 185ºF (85ºC). If it's not, use the Sauté function to warm to 185.
4. After it reaches 185ºF (85ºC), unplug Instant Pot, remove inner pot, and cool. You can place on cooling rack and let it slowly cool. If in a hurry, submerge the base of the pot in cool water. Cool milk to 110ºF (43ºC).
5. When mixture reaches 110, stir in the ¼ cup of yogurt. Lock the lid in place and move vent to sealing.
6. Press Yogurt. Use the Adjust button until the screen says 8:00. This will now incubate for 8 hours.
7. After 8 hours (when the cycle is finished), chill yogurt, or go immediately to straining in step 8.
8. After chilling, or following the 8 hours, strain the yogurt using a nut milk bag. This will give it the consistency of Greek yogurt.

**Per Serving**

calories: 141 | fat: 5g | protein: 10g | carbs: 14g | sugars: 1g | fiber: 0g | sodium: 145mg

# Smoked Salmon and Asparagus Quiche Cups

Prep time: 15 minutes | Cook time: 15 minutes | Serves 2

Nonstick cooking spray
2 tablespoons finely chopped onion
3 ounces (85 g) smoked salmon (skinless and boneless), chopped
3 large eggs
¼ teaspoon dried dill

4 asparagus spears, cut into ½-inch pieces

2 tablespoons 2% milk
Pinch ground white pepper

1. Pour 1½ cups of water into the electric pressure cooker and insert a wire rack or trivet.
2. Lightly spray the bottom and sides of the ramekins with nonstick cooking spray. Divide the asparagus, onion, and salmon between the ramekins.
3. In a measuring cup with a spout, whisk together the eggs, milk, dill, and white pepper. Pour half of the egg mixture into each ramekin. Loosely cover the ramekins with aluminum foil.
4. Carefully place the ramekins inside the pot on the rack.
5. Close and lock the lid of the pressure cooker. Set the valve to sealing.
6. Cook on high pressure for 15 minutes.
7. When the cooking is complete, hit Cancel and quick release the pressure.
8. Once the pin drops, unlock and remove the lid.
9. Carefully remove the ramekins from the pot. Cool, covered, for 5 minutes.
10. Run a small silicone spatula or a knife around the edge of each ramekin. Invert each quiche onto a small plate and serve.

**Per Serving**
calories: 180 | fat: 9g | protein: 20g | carbs: 3g | sugars: 1g | fiber: 1g | sodium: 646mg

# Southwestern Egg Casserole

Prep time: 10 minutes | Cook time: 20 minutes | Serves 12

1 cup water
½ cup flour
⅛ teaspoon salt
2 cups fat-free cottage cheese
1½ cups shredded 75%-less-fat sharp Cheddar cheese
¼ cup no-trans-fat tub margarine, melted
2 (4-ounce / 113-g) cans chopped green chilies

2½ cups egg substitute
1 teaspoon baking powder
⅛ teaspoon pepper

1. Place the steam rack into the bottom of the inner pot and pour in 1 cup of water.
2. Grease a round springform pan that will fit into the inner pot of the Instant Pot.
3. Combine the egg substitute, flour, baking powder, salt and pepper in a mixing bowl. It will be lumpy.
4. Stir in the cheese, margarine, and green chilies then pour into the springform pan.
5. Place the springform pan onto the steam rack, close the lid, and secure to the locking position. Be sure the vent is turned to sealing. Set for 20 minutes on Manual at high pressure.
6. Let the pressure release naturally.
7. Carefully remove the springform pan with the handles of the steam rack and allow to stand 10 minutes before cutting and serving.

**Per Serving**
calories: 130 | fat: 4g | protein: 14g | carbs: 9g | sugars: 1g | fiber: 1g | sodium: 450mg

# Shakshuka with Swiss Chard

**Prep time: 15 minutes | Cook time: 10 minutes | Serves 4**

4 ounces (113 g) Swiss chard (about 4 large stems and leaves)

2 tablespoons extra-virgin olive oil

½ teaspoon kosher salt

½ tablespoon Italian seasoning

1½ cups tomato-based pasta sauce

1 tablespoon chopped fresh parsley

½ medium onion, chopped

½ teaspoon freshly ground black pepper

2 teaspoons minced garlic

4 large eggs

2 tablespoons freshly grated Parmesan cheese

1. Separate the stems from the leaves of the Swiss chard. Finely chop the stems; you'll need about ½ cup. Stack the leaves, slice into thin strips, then chop. Set aside.
2. Set the electric pressure cooker to the Sauté setting. When the pot is hot, pour in the olive oil.
3. Add the Swiss chard stems, onion, salt, pepper, and Italian seasoning to the pot, and sauté for 3 to 5 minutes or until the vegetables begin to soften.
4. Add the Swiss chard leaves and garlic, and sauté for 2 more minutes.
5. Hit Cancel. Add the pasta sauce and let the pot cool for 5 minutes.
6. Make 4 evenly spaced indentations in the sauce mixture. Carefully crack an egg into a custard cup, then pour it into one of the indentations. Repeat with the remaining eggs. (Note you can crack the eggs directly into the pot, but the whites will spread out more and the eggs won't look as nice.)
7. Close and lock the lid of the pressure cooker. Set the valve to sealing.
8. Select low pressure and set the timer for 0 minutes.
9. When the cooking is complete, hit Cancel and quick release the pressure.
10. Once the pin drops, unlock and remove the lid.
11. Sprinkle with parsley and Parmesan, and serve immediately.

**Per Serving**

calories: 182 | fat: 12g | protein: 8g | carbs: 11g | sugars: 6g | fiber: 3g | sodium: 851mg

# Tropical Steel Cut Oats

**Prep time: 5 minutes | Cook time: 5 minutes | Serves 4**

1 cup steel cut oats

2 cups coconut water or water

¾ cup frozen mango chunks

Ground cinnamon

1 cup unsweetened almond milk

¾ cup frozen chopped peaches

1 (2-inch) vanilla bean, scraped (seeds and pod)

¼ cup chopped unsalted macadamia nuts

1. In the electric pressure cooker, combine the oats, almond milk, coconut water, peaches, mango chunks, and vanilla bean seeds and pod. Stir well.
2. Close and lock the lid of the pressure cooker. Set the valve to sealing.
3. Cook on high pressure for 5 minutes.
4. When the cooking is complete, allow the pressure to release naturally for 10 minutes, then quick release any remaining pressure. Hit Cancel.
5. Once the pin drops, unlock and remove the lid.
6. Discard the vanilla bean pod and stir well.
7. Spoon the oats into 4 bowls. Top each serving with a sprinkle of cinnamon and 1 tablespoon of the macadamia nuts.

**Per Serving (¾ cup)**

calories: 127 | fat: 7g | protein: 2g | carbs: 14g | sugars: 8g | fiber: 3g | sodium: 167mg

# Blueberry Oat Mini Muffins

**Prep time: 12 minutes | Cook time: 10 minutes | Serves 7**

½ cup rolled oats
¼ cup whole wheat pastry flour or white whole wheat flour
½ tablespoon baking powder
⅛ teaspoon kosher salt
½ cup plain Greek yogurt
2 teaspoons extra-virgin olive oil
½ teaspoon ground cardamom or ground cinnamon
2 large eggs
2 tablespoons pure maple syrup
½ teaspoon vanilla extract
½ cup frozen blueberries (preferably small wild blueberries)

1. In a large bowl, stir together the oats, flour, baking powder, cardamom, and salt.
2. In a medium bowl, whisk together the eggs, yogurt, maple syrup, oil, and vanilla.
3. Add the egg mixture to oat mixture and stir just until combined. Gently fold in the blueberries.
4. Scoop the batter into each cup of the egg bite mold.
5. Pour 1 cup of water into the electric pressure cooker. Place the egg bite mold on the wire rack and carefully lower it into the pot.
6. Close and lock the lid of the pressure cooker. Set the valve to sealing.
7. Cook on high pressure for 10 minutes.
8. When the cooking is complete, allow the pressure to release naturally for 10 minutes, then quick release any remaining pressure. Hit Cancel.
9. Lift the wire rack out of the pot and place on a cooling rack for 5 minutes. Invert the mold onto the cooling rack to release the muffins.
10. Serve the muffins warm or refrigerate or freeze.

**Per Serving**
calories: 117 | fat: 4g | protein: 5g | carbs: 15g | sugars: 4g | fiber: 2g | sodium: 89mg

# Cinnamon French Toast

**Prep time: 10 minutes | Cook time: 20 minutes | Serves 8**

3 eggs
2 tablespoons maple syrup
2 teaspoons vanilla extract
**Pinch salt**
2 cups low-fat milk
15 drops liquid stevia
2 teaspoons cinnamon
16 ounces (454 g) whole wheat bread, cubed and left out overnight to go stale
1½ cups water

1. In a medium bowl, whisk together the eggs, milk, maple syrup, stevia, vanilla, cinnamon, and salt. Stir in the cubes of whole wheat bread.
2. You will need a 7-inch round baking pan for this. Spray the inside with nonstick spray, then pour the bread mixture into the pan.
3. Place the trivet in the bottom of the inner pot, then pour in the water.
4. Make foil sling and insert it onto the trivet. Carefully place the 7-inch pan on top of the foil sling/trivet.
5. Secure the lid to the locked position, then make sure the vent is turned to sealing.
6. Press the Manual button and use the "+/-" button to set the Instant Pot for 20 minutes.
7. When cook time is up, let the Instant Pot release naturally for 5 minutes, then quick release the rest.

**Per Serving**
calories: 75 | fat: 3g | protein: 4g | carbs: 7g | sugars: 6g | fiber: 0g | sodium: 74mg

## Baked Eggs

**Prep time: 15 minutes | Cook time: 20 minutes | Serves 8**

1 cup water
1 cup reduced-fat buttermilk baking mix
2 teaspoons chopped onion
½ cup grated reduced-fat Cheddar cheese
1¼ cups egg substitute

2 tablespoons no-trans-fat tub margarine, melted
1½ cups fat-free cottage cheese
1 teaspoon dried parsley
1 egg, slightly beaten
1 cup fat-free milk

1. Place the steam rack into the bottom of the inner pot and pour in 1 cup of water.
2. Grease a round springform pan that will fit into the inner pot of the Instant Pot.
3. Pour melted margarine into springform pan.
4. Mix together buttermilk baking mix, cottage cheese, onion, parsley, cheese, egg, egg substitute, and milk in large mixing bowl.
5. Pour mixture over melted margarine. Stir slightly to distribute margarine.
6. Place the springform pan onto the steam rack, close the lid, and secure to the locking position. Be sure the vent is turned to sealing. Set for 20 minutes on Manual at high pressure.
7. Let the pressure release naturally.
8. Carefully remove the springform pan with the handles of the steam rack and allow to stand 10 minutes before cutting and serving.

**Per Serving**
calories: 155 | fat: 5g | protein: 12g | carbs: 15g | sugars: 4g | fiber: 0g | sodium: 460mg

## Easy Quiche

**Prep time: 15 minutes | Cook time: 25 minutes | Serves 6**

1 cup water
¼ cup chopped mushroom, optional
3 ounces (85 g) 75%-less-fat Cheddar cheese, shredded
2 tablespoons bacon bits, chopped ham or browned sausage
4 eggs
1½ cups fat-free milk
1 tablespoon trans-fat-free tub margarine

¼ cup chopped onion

¼ teaspoons salt
½ cup whole wheat flour

1. Pour water into Instant Pot and place the steam rack inside.
2. Spray a 6-inch round cake pan with nonstick spray.
3. Sprinkle the onion, mushroom, shredded Cheddar, and meat around in the cake pan.
4. Combine remaining ingredients in medium bowl. Pour over meat and vegetables mixture.
5. Place the cake pan onto the steam rack, close the lid and secure to the locking position. Be sure the vent is turned to sealing. Set for 25 minutes on Manual at high pressure.
6. Let the pressure release naturally.
7. Carefully remove the cake pan with the handles of the steam rack and allow to stand 10 minutes before cutting and serving.

**Per Serving**
calories: 128 | fat: 5g | protein: 11g | carbs: 10g | sugars: 2g | fiber: 1g | sodium: 302mg

# Potato-Bacon Gratin

**Prep time: 20 minutes | Cook time: 40 minutes | Serves 8**

1 tablespoon olive oil
1 clove garlic, minced
6 ounces (170 g) Canadian bacon slices, divided
1 cup lower-sodium, lower-fat chicken broth

1 (6-ounce / 170-g) bag fresh spinach
4 large potatoes, peeled or unpeeled, divided
5 ounces (142 g) reduced-fat grated Swiss Cheddar, divided

1. Set the Instant Pot to Sauté and pour in the olive oil. Cook the spinach and garlic in olive oil just until spinach is wilted (5 minutes or less). Turn off the instant pot.
2. Cut potatoes into thin slices about ¼ inch thick.
3. In a springform pan that will fit into the inner pot of your Instant Pot, spray it with nonstick spray then layer ⅓ the potatoes, half the bacon, ⅓ the cheese, and half the wilted spinach.
4. Repeat layers ending with potatoes. Reserve ⅓ cheese for later.
5. Pour chicken broth over all.
6. Wipe the bottom of your Instant Pot to soak up any remaining oil, then add in 2 cups of water and the steam rack. Place the springform pan on top.
7. Close the lid and secure to the locking position. Be sure the vent is turned to sealing. Set for 35 minutes on Manual at high pressure.
8. Perform a quick release.
9. Top with the remaining cheese, then allow to stand 10 minutes before removing from the Instant Pot, cutting and serving.

**Per Serving**
calories: 220 | fat: 7g | protein: 14g | carbs: 28g | sugars: 2g | fiber: 3g | sodium: 415mg

# Shredded Potato Omelet

**Prep time: 15 minutes | Cook time: 20 minutes | Serves 6**

3 slices bacon, cooked and crumbled
¼ cup minced onion
1 cup egg substitute
¼ teaspoon salt
1 cup 75%-less-fat shredded Cheddar cheese

2 cups shredded cooked potatoes
¼ cup minced green bell pepper
¼ cup fat-free milk
⅛ teaspoon black pepper
1 cup water

1. With nonstick cooking spray, spray the inside of a round baking dish that will fit in your Instant Pot inner pot.
2. Sprinkle the bacon, potatoes, onion, and bell pepper around the bottom of the baking dish.
3. Mix together the egg substitute, milk, salt, and pepper in mixing bowl. Pour over potato mixture.
4. Top with cheese.
5. Add water, place the steam rack into the bottom of the inner pot and then place the round baking dish on top.
6. Close the lid and secure to the locking position. Be sure the vent is turned to sealing. Set for 20 minutes on Manual at high pressure.
7. Let the pressure release naturally.
8. Carefully remove the baking dish with the handles of the steam rack and allow to stand 10 minutes before cutting and serving.

**Per Serving**
calories: 130 | fat: 3g | protein: 12g | carbs: 13g | sugars: 2g | fiber: 2g | sodium: 415mg

# Coddled Huevos Rancheros



**Prep time: 5 minutes | Cook time: 10 minutes | Serves 2**

2 teaspoons unsalted butter
1 cup drained cooked black beans, or ⅔ (15-ounce / 425-g) can black beans, rinsed and drained
2 (7-inch) corn or whole-wheat tortillas, warmed
2 cups shredded romaine lettuce
2 tablespoons grated Cotija cheese

4 large eggs

½ cup chunky tomato salsa (such as Pace brand)
1 tablespoon chopped fresh cilantro

1. Pour 1 cup water into the Instant Pot and place a long-handled silicone steam rack into the pot. (If you don't have the long-handled rack, use the wire metal steam rack and a homemade sling)
2. Coat each of four 4-ounce (113-g) ramekins with ½ teaspoon butter. Crack an egg into each ramekin. Place the ramekins on the steam rack in the pot.
3. Secure the lid and set the Pressure Release to Sealing. Select the Steam setting and set the cooking time for 3 minutes at low pressure. (The pot will take about 5 minutes to come up to pressure before the cooking program begins.)
4. While the eggs are cooking, in a small saucepan over low heat, warm the beans for about 5 minutes, stirring occasionally. Cover the saucepan and remove from the heat. (Alternatively, warm the beans in a covered bowl in a microwave for 1 minute. Leave the beans covered until ready to serve.)
5. When the cooking program ends, let the pressure release naturally for 5 minutes, then move the Pressure Release to Venting to release any remaining steam. Open the pot and, wearing heat-resistant mitts, grasp the handles of the steam rack and carefully lift it out of the pot.
6. Place a warmed tortilla on each plate and spoon ½ cup of the beans onto each tortilla. Run a knife around the inside edge of each ramekin to loosen the egg and unmold two eggs onto the beans on each tortilla. Spoon the salsa over the eggs and top with the lettuce, cilantro, and cheese. Serve right away.

**Per Serving**
calories: 383 | fat: 16g | protein: 23g | carbs: 35g | sugars: 5g | fiber: 8g | sodium: 592mg

# Cranberry Almond Grits

**Prep time: 10 minutes | Cook time: 10 minutes | Serves 5**

¾ cup stone-ground grits or polenta (not instant)
½ cup unsweetened dried cranberries
1 tablespoon unsalted butter or ghee (optional)
1 tablespoon half-and-half

Pinch kosher salt

¼ cup sliced almonds, toasted

1. In the electric pressure cooker, stir together the grits, cranberries, salt, and 3 cups of water.
2. Close and lock the lid. Set the valve to sealing.
3. Cook on high pressure for 10 minutes.
4. When the cooking is complete, hit Cancel and quick release the pressure.
5. Once the pin drops, unlock and remove the lid.
6. Add the butter (if using) and half-and-half. Stir until the mixture is creamy, adding more half-and-half if necessary.
7. Spoon into serving bowls and sprinkle with almonds.

**Per Serving (½ cup)**
calories: 218 | fat: 10g | protein: 5g | carbs: 32g | sugars: 7g | fiber: 4g | sodium: 28mg

# Egg Bites with Sausage and Peppers

**Prep time: 5 minutes | Cook time: 15 minutes | Serves 7**

**4 large eggs**

**¼ cup vegan cream cheese (such as Tofutti brand) or cream cheese**

**¼ teaspoon fine sea salt**

**¼ teaspoon freshly ground black pepper**

**3 ounces (85 g) lean turkey sausage, cooked and crumbled, or 1 vegetarian sausage (such as Beyond Meat brand), cooked and diced**

**½ red bell pepper, seeded and chopped**

**2 green onions, white and green parts, minced, plus more for garnish (optional)**

**¼ cup vegan cheese shreds or shredded sharp Cheddar cheese**

1. In a blender, combine the eggs, cream cheese, salt, and pepper. Blend on medium speed for about 20 seconds, just until combined. Add the sausage, bell pepper, and green onions and pulse for 1 second once or twice. You want to mix in the solid ingredients without grinding them up very much.

2. Pour 1 cup water into the Instant Pot. Generously grease a 7-cup egg-bite mold or seven 2-ounce (57-g) silicone baking cups with butter or coconut oil, making sure to coat each cup well. Place the prepared mold or cups on a long-handled silicone steam rack. (If you don't have the long-handled rack, use the wire metal steam rack and a homemade sling)

3. Pour ¼ cup of the egg mixture into each prepared mold or cup. Holding the handles of the steam rack, carefully lower the egg bites into the pot.

4. Secure the lid and set the Pressure Release to Sealing. Select the Steam setting and set the cooking time for 8 minutes at low pressure. (The pot will take about 5 minutes to come up to pressure before the cooking program begins.)

5. When the cooking program ends, let the pressure release naturally for 5 minutes, then move the Pressure Release to Venting to release any remaining steam. Open the pot. The egg muffins will have puffed up quite a bit during cooking, but they will deflate and settle as they cool. Wearing heat-resistant mitts, grasp the handles of the steam rack and carefully lift the egg bites out of the pot. Sprinkle the egg bites with the cheese, then let them cool for about 5 minutes, until the cheese has fully melted and you are able to handle the mold or cups comfortably.

6. Pull the sides of the egg mold or cups away from the egg bites, running a butter knife around the edge of each bite to loosen if necessary. Transfer the egg bites to plates, garnish with more green onions (if desired), and serve warm. To store, let cool to room temperature, transfer to an airtight container, and refrigerate for up to 3 days; reheat gently in the microwave for about 1 minute before serving.

**Per Serving**

**calories: 112 | fat: 8g | protein: 8g | carbs: 3g | sugars: 0g | fiber: 0g | sodium: 297mg**

# Best Steel-Cut Oats



1 cup steel-cut oats

1 cup unsweetened almond milk

**Pinch salt**

½ teaspoon vanilla extract

¼ cup raisins

1 teaspoon ground cinnamon

**Sweetener of choice, optional**

2 cups water

1 cinnamon stick

¼ cup dried cherries

¼ cup toasted almonds

1. Add all ingredients to the inner pot of the Instant Pot except the toasted almonds and sweetener.
2. Secure the lid and make sure the vent is turned to sealing. Cook 3 minutes on high, using Manual function.
3. Let the pressure release naturally.
4. Remove cinnamon stick.
5. Add almonds, and sweetener if desired, and serve.

**Per Serving**

calories: 276 | fat: 7g | protein: 9g | carbs: 46g | sugars: 9g | fiber: 7g | sodium: 53mg

# Carrot Cake Oatmeal



2 tablespoons vegan buttery spread or unsalted butter

1½ cups steel-cut oats (gluten-free, if desired)

4½ cups water

2 teaspoons ground cinnamon, plus more for serving

¾ teaspoon ground ginger

½ teaspoon fine sea salt

¾ cup chopped toasted walnuts

**Sugar-free maple-flavored syrup, for serving (optional)**

8 ounces (227 g) carrots, finely grated

½ teaspoon ground nutmeg

1 ripe banana, peeled and mashed

1. Select the Sauté setting on the Instant Pot and melt the buttery spread. Add the oats and cook, stirring often, for about 5 minutes, until the oats are aromatic and lightly toasted. Stir in the water, carrots, cinnamon, ginger, nutmeg, and salt, using a wooden spoon to nudge any browned bits from the bottom of the pot and making sure all of the oats are submerged in the liquid.
2. Secure the lid and set the Pressure Release to Sealing. Press the Cancel button to reset the cooking program, then select the Porridge or Manual setting and set the cooking time for 12 minutes at high pressure. (The pot will take about 10 minutes to come up to pressure before the cooking program begins.)
3. When the cooking program ends, let the pressure release naturally for at least 10 minutes, then move the Pressure Release to Venting to release any remaining steam. Open the pot and stir in the banana and any extra liquid sitting on top of the oatmeal.
4. Ladle the oatmeal into bowls and sprinkle with the nuts and additional cinnamon. Pass the syrup, if desired, when serving.

**Per Serving**

calories: 321 | fat: 17g | protein: 8g | carbs: 38g | sugars: 4g | fiber: 7g | sodium: 255mg

# Coddled Eggs and Smoked Salmon Toasts

**Prep time: 5 minutes | Cook time: 10 minutes | Serves 4**

2 teaspoons unsalted butter

4 slices gluten-free or whole-grain rye bread

4 ounces (113 g) cold-smoked salmon, or 1 medium avocado, pitted, peeled, and sliced

2 radishes, thinly sliced

1 tablespoon chopped fresh chives

4 large eggs

½ cup plain 2 percent Greek yogurt

1 Persian cucumber, thinly sliced

¼ teaspoon freshly ground black pepper

1. Pour 1 cup water into the Instant Pot and place a long-handled silicone steam rack into the pot. (If you don't have the long-handled rack, use the wire metal steam rack and a homemade sling)
2. Coat each of four 4-ounce (113-g) ramekins with ½ teaspoon butter. Crack an egg into each ramekin. Place the ramekins on the steam rack in the pot.
3. Secure the lid and set the Pressure Release to Sealing. Select the Steam setting and set the cooking time for 3 minutes at low pressure. (The pot will take about 5 minutes to come up to pressure before the cooking program begins.)
4. While eggs are cooking, toast the bread in a toaster until golden brown. Spread the yogurt onto the toasted slices, put the toasts onto plates, and then top each toast with the smoked salmon, radishes, and cucumber.
5. When the cooking program ends, let the pressure release naturally for 5 minutes, then move the Pressure Release to Venting to release any remaining steam. Open the pot and, wearing heat-resistant mitts, grasp the handles of the steam rack and lift it out of the pot.
6. Run a knife around the inside edge of each ramekin to loosen the egg and unmold one egg onto each toast. Sprinkle the chives and pepper on top and serve right away.

**Per Serving**

calories: 275 | fat: 12g | protein: 21g | carbs: 21g | sugars: 4g | fiber: 5g | sodium: 431mg

# Breakfast Farro with Berries and Walnuts

**Prep time: 8 minutes | Cook time: 10 minutes | Serves 6**

1 cup farro, rinsed and drained

¼ teaspoon kosher salt

1 teaspoon ground cinnamon

1½ cups fresh blueberries, raspberries, or strawberries (or a combination)

6 tablespoons chopped walnuts

1 cup unsweetened almond milk

½ teaspoon pure vanilla extract

1 tablespoon pure maple syrup

1. In the electric pressure cooker, combine the farro, almond milk, 1 cup of water, salt, vanilla, cinnamon, and maple syrup.
2. Close and lock the lid. Set the valve to sealing.
3. Cook on high pressure for 10 minutes.
4. When the cooking is complete, allow the pressure to release naturally for 10 minutes, then quick release any remaining pressure. Hit Cancel.
5. Once the pin drops, unlock and remove the lid.
6. Stir the farro. Spoon into bowls and top each serving with ¼ cup of berries and 1 tablespoon of walnuts.

**Per Serving (⅓ cup)**

calories: 189 | fat: 5g | protein: 5g | carbs: 32g | sugars: 6g | fiber: 3g | sodium: 111mg

# Instant Pot Hard-Boiled Eggs

**Prep time: 10 minutes | Cook time: 5 minutes | Serves 7**

1 cup water

6 to 8 eggs

1. Pour the water into the inner pot. Place the eggs in a steamer basket or rack that came with pot.
2. Close the lid and secure to the locking position. Be sure the vent is turned to sealing. Set for 5 minutes on Manual at high pressure. (It takes about 5 minutes for pressure to build and then 5 minutes to cook.)
3. Let pressure naturally release for 5 minutes, then do quick pressure release.
4. Place hot eggs into cool water to halt cooking process. You can peel cooled eggs immediately or refrigerate unpeeled.

**Per Serving**

calories: 72 | fat: 5g | protein: 6g | carbs: 0g | sugars: 0g | fiber: 0g | sodium: 71mg

# Free Apple Cinnamon Cake

**Prep time: 10 minutes | Cook time: 50 minutes | Serves 8**

2 cups almond flour
1½ teaspoons ground cinnamon
½ teaspoon fine sea salt
2 large eggs
1 small apple, chopped into small pieces

½ cup Lakanto Monkfruit Sweetener Golden
1 teaspoon baking powder
½ cup plain 2 percent Greek yogurt
½ teaspoon pure vanilla extract

1. Pour 1 cup water into the Instant Pot. Line the base of a 7 by 3-inch round cake pan with parchment paper. Butter the sides of the pan and the parchment or coat with nonstick cooking spray.
2. In a medium bowl, whisk together the almond flour, sweetener, cinnamon, baking powder, and salt. In a smaller bowl, whisk together the yogurt, eggs, and vanilla until no streaks of yolk remain. Add the wet mixture to the dry mixture and stir just until the dry ingredients are evenly moistened, then fold in the apple. The batter will be very thick.
3. Transfer the batter to the prepared pan and, using a rubber spatula, spread it in an even layer. Cover the pan tightly with aluminum foil. Place the pan on a long-handled silicone steam rack, then, holding the handles of the steam rack, lower it into the Instant Pot. (If you don't have the long-handled rack, use the wire metal steam rack and a homemade sling)
4. Secure the lid and set the Pressure Release to Sealing. Select the Manual setting and set the cooking time for 40 minutes at high pressure. (The pot will take about 10 minutes to come up to pressure before the cooking program begins.)
5. When the cooking program ends, let the pressure release naturally for 10 minutes, then move the Pressure Release to Venting to release any remaining steam. Open the pot and, wearing heat-resistant mitts, grasp the handles of the steam rack and lift it out of the pot. Uncover the pan, taking care not to get burned by the steam or to drip condensation onto the cake. Let the cake cool in the pan on a cooling rack for about 5 minutes.
6. Run a butter knife around the edge of the pan to loosen the cake from the pan sides. Invert the cake onto the rack, lift off the pan, and peel off the parchment. Let cool for 15 minutes, then invert the cake onto a serving plate. Cut into eight wedges and serve.

**Per Serving**

calories: 219 | fat: 16g | protein: 9g | carbs: 20g | sugars: 8g | fiber: 16g | sodium: 154mg

# Breakfast Millet with Nuts and Strawberries

**Prep time: 5 minutes | Cook time: 30 minutes | Serves 8**

**2 tablespoons coconut oil or unsalted butter**
**1½ cups millet**
**2⅔ cups water**
**½ teaspoon fine sea salt**
**1 cup unsweetened almond milk or other nondairy milk**
**1 cup chopped toasted pecans, almonds, or peanuts**
**4 cups sliced strawberries**

1. Select the Sauté setting on the Instant Pot and melt the oil. Add the millet and cook for 4 minutes, until aromatic. Stir in the water and salt, making sure all of the grains are submerged in the liquid.
2. Secure the lid and set the Pressure Release to Sealing. Press the Cancel button to reset the cooking program, then select the Porridge or Manual setting and set the cooking time for 12 minutes at high pressure. (The pot will take about 10 minutes to come up to pressure before the cooking program begins.)
3. When the cooking program ends, let the pressure release naturally for 10 minutes, then move the Pressure Release to Venting to release any remaining steam. Open the pot and use a fork to fluff and stir the millet.
4. Spoon the millet into bowls and top each serving with 2 tablespoons of the almond milk, then sprinkle with the nuts and top with the strawberries. Serve warm.

**Per Serving**
calories: 270 | fat: 13g | protein: 6g | carbs: 35g | sugars: 4g | fiber: 6g | sodium: 151mg

# Poached Eggs

**Prep time: 5 minutes | Cook time: 5 minutes | Serves 4**

**Nonstick cooking spray**
**4 large eggs**

1. Lightly spray 4 cups of a 7-count silicone egg bite mold with nonstick cooking spray. Crack each egg into a sprayed cup.
2. Pour 1 cup of water into the electric pressure cooker. Place the egg bite mold on the wire rack and carefully lower it into the pot.
3. Close and lock the lid of the pressure cooker. Set the valve to sealing.
4. Cook on high pressure for 5 minutes.
5. When the cooking is complete, hit Cancel and quick release the pressure.
6. Once the pin drops, unlock and remove the lid.
7. Run a small rubber spatula or spoon around each egg and carefully remove it from the mold. The white should be cooked, but the yolk should be runny.
8. Serve immediately.

**Per Serving**
calories: 78 | fat: 5g | protein: 6g | carbs: 1g | sugars: 0g | fiber: 0g | sodium: 62mgGrain

# Greek Frittata with Peppers, Kale, and Feta

**Prep time: 5 minutes | Cook time: 45 minutes | Serves 6**

8 large eggs

Fine sea salt, to taste

2 cups firmly packed finely shredded kale or baby kale leaves

1 (12-ounce / 340-g) jar roasted red peppers, drained and cut into ¼ by 2-inch strips

2 green onions, white and green parts, thinly sliced

1 tablespoon chopped fresh dill

6 cups loosely packed mixed baby greens

2 tablespoons extra-virgin olive oil

½ cup plain 2 percent Greek yogurt

Freshly ground black pepper, to taste

⅓ cup crumbled feta cheese

¾ cup cherry or grape tomatoes, halved

1. Pour 1½ cups water into the Instant Pot. Lightly butter a 7-cup round heatproof glass dish or coat with nonstick cooking spray.
2. In a bowl, whisk together the eggs, yogurt, ¼ teaspoon salt, and ¼ teaspoon pepper until well blended, then stir in the kale, roasted peppers, green onions, dill, and feta cheese.
3. Pour the egg mixture into the prepared dish and cover tightly with aluminum foil. Place the dish on a long-handled silicone steam rack, then, holding the handles of the steam rack, lower it into the Instant Pot. (If you don't have the long-handled rack, use the wire metal steam rack and a homemade sling)
4. Secure the lid and set the Pressure Release to Sealing. Select the Manual setting and set the cooking time for 30 minutes at high pressure. (The pot will take about 15 minutes to come up to pressure before the cooking program begins.)
5. When the cooking program ends, let the pressure release naturally for 10 minutes, then move the Pressure Release to Venting to release any remaining steam. Open the pot and let the frittata sit for a minute or two, until it deflates and settles into its dish. Then, wearing heat-resistant mitts, grasp the handles of the steam rack and lift it out of the pot. Uncover the dish, taking care not to get burned by the steam or to drip condensation onto the frittata. Let the frittata sit for 10 minutes, giving it time to reabsorb any liquid and set up.
6. In a medium bowl, toss together the mixed greens, tomatoes, and olive oil. Taste and adjust the seasoning with salt and pepper, if needed.
7. Cut the frittata into six wedges and serve warm, with the salad alongside.

**Per Serving (frittata only)**
calories: 227 | fat: 13g | protein: 18g | carbs: 8g | sugars: 2g | fiber: 1g | sodium: 153mg

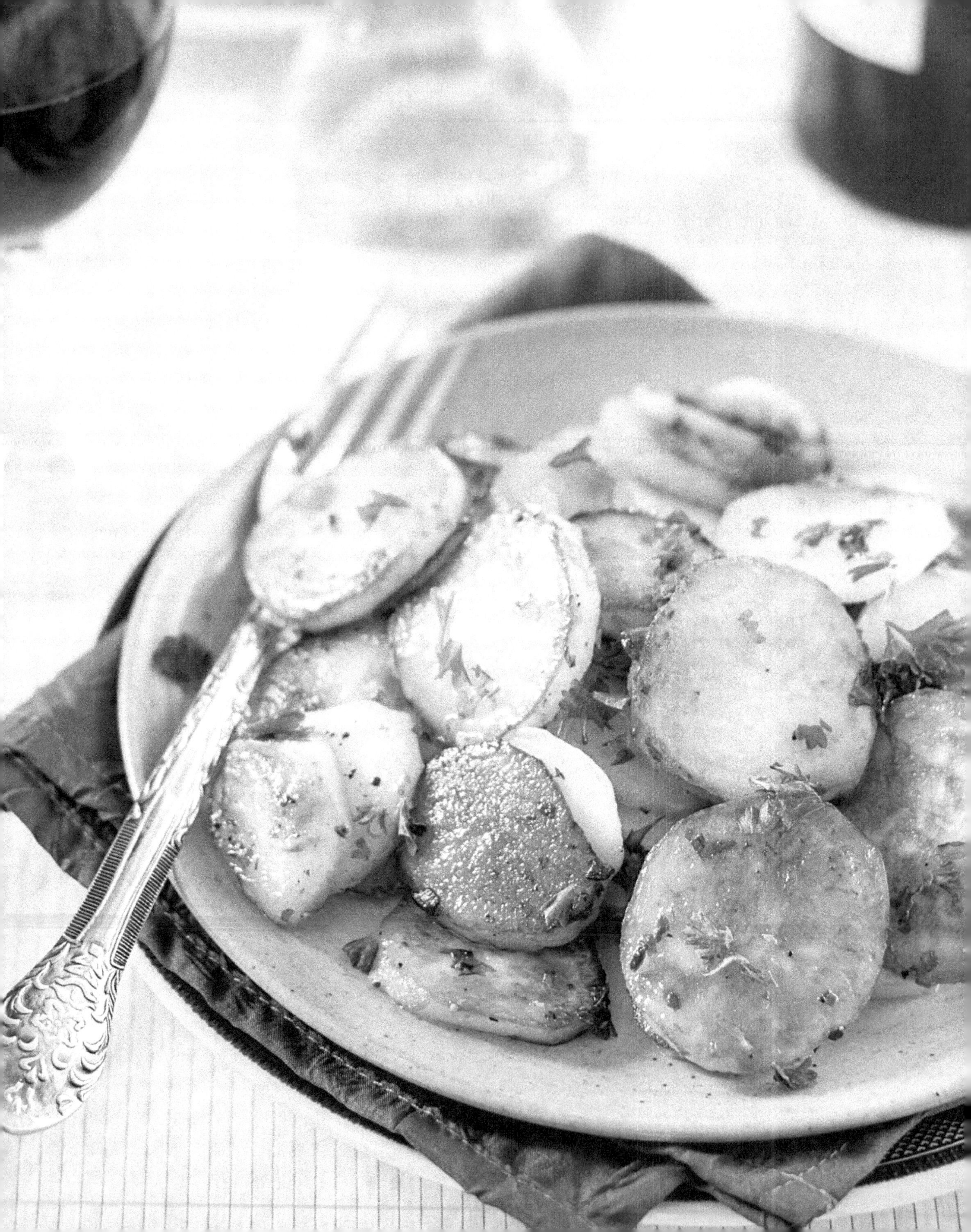

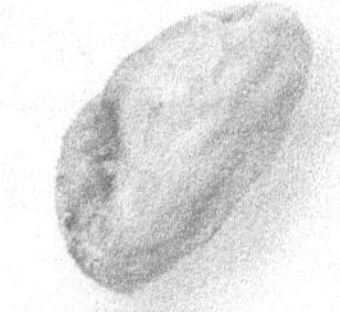


25   Hummus   30

26   Candied Pecans   30

27   Ground Turkey Lettuce Cups   31

28   7-Layer Dip   32

29   Lemon Artichokes   33

30   Instant Popcorn   33

31   Blackberry Baked Brie   33

32   Creamy Spinach Dip   34

33   Smoky Deviled Eggs   34

34   Creamy Jalapeño Chicken Dip   35

35   Green Goddess White Bean Dip   35

36   Porcupine Meatballs   36

37   Buffalo Chicken Dip   36

38   Artichoke Spinach Dip   37


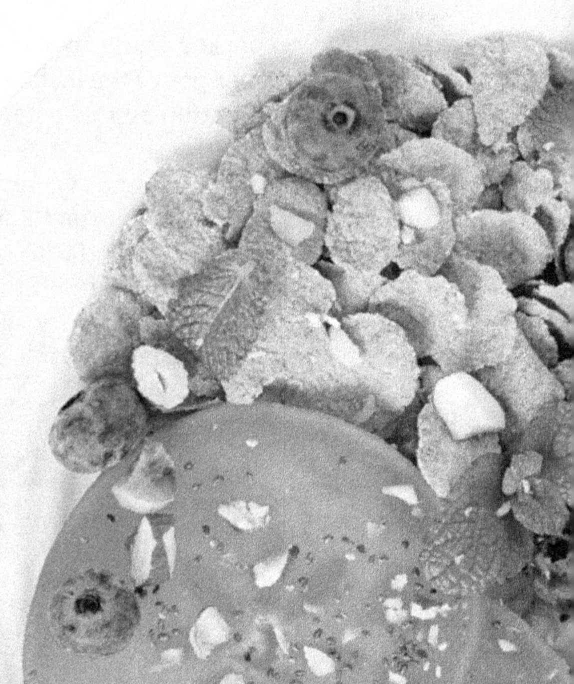

# Hummus



1 cup dry garbanzo beans (chickpeas)
2 tablespoons fresh lemon juice
3 cloves garlic, minced
2 teaspoons olive oil
Pinch cayenne pepper

4 cups water
¼ cup chopped onion
½ cup tahini (sesame paste)
2 teaspoons cumin
½ teaspoon salt, optional

1. Place garbanzo beans and 4 cups water into inner pot of Instant Pot. Secure lid and make sure vent is set to sealing.
2. Cook garbanzo beans and water for 40 minutes using the Manual high pressure setting.
3. When cooking time is up, let the pressure release naturally.
4. Test the garbanzos. If still firm, cook using Slow Cook function until they are soft.
5. Drain the garbanzo beans, but save ½ cup of the cooking liquid.
6. Combine the garbanzos, lemon juice, onion, garlic, tahini, oil, cumin, pepper, and optional salt in a blender or food processor.
7. Purée until smooth, adding chickpea liquid as needed to thin the purée. Taste and adjust seasonings accordingly.

**Per Serving**
calories: 200 | fat: 11g | protein: 8g | carbs: 20g | sugars: 3g | fiber: 4g | sodium: 16mg

# Candied Pecans



4 cups raw pecans
½ cup plus 1 tablespoon water, divided
1 teaspoon cinnamon
⅛ teaspoon ground ginger

1½ teaspoons liquid stevia
1 teaspoon vanilla extract
¼ teaspoon nutmeg
⅛ teaspoon sea salt

1. Place the raw pecans, liquid stevia, 1 tablespoon water, vanilla, cinnamon, nutmeg, ground ginger, and sea salt into the inner pot of the Instant Pot.
2. Press the Sauté button on the Instant Pot and sauté the pecans and other ingredients until the pecans are soft.
3. Pour in the ½ cup water and secure the lid to the locked position. Set the vent to sealing.
4. Press Manual and set the Instant Pot for 15 minutes.
5. Preheat the oven to 350ºF (180ºC).
6. When cooking time is up, turn off the Instant Pot, then do a quick release.
7. Spread the pecans onto a greased, lined baking sheet.
8. Bake the pecans for 5 minutes or less in the oven, checking on them frequently so they do not burn.

**Per Serving**
calories: 275 | fat: 28g | protein: 4g | carbs: 6g | sugars: 2g | fiber: 4g | sodium: 20mg

# Ground Turkey Lettuce Cups

**Prep time: 5 minutes | Cook time: 30 minutes | Serves 8**

3 tablespoons water
2 tablespoons soy sauce, tamari, or coconut aminos
3 tablespoons fresh lime juice
2 teaspoons Sriracha, plus more for serving
2 tablespoons cold-pressed avocado oil
2 teaspoons toasted sesame oil
4 garlic cloves, minced
1-inch piece fresh ginger, peeled and minced
2 carrots, diced
2 celery stalks, diced
1 yellow onion, diced
2 pounds (907 g) 93 percent lean ground turkey
½ teaspoon fine sea salt
2 (8-ounce / 227-g) cans sliced water chestnuts, drained and chopped
1 tablespoon cornstarch
2 hearts romaine lettuce or 2 heads butter lettuce, leaves separated
½ cup roasted cashews (whole or halves and pieces), chopped
1 cup loosely packed fresh cilantro leaves

1.  In a small bowl, combine the water, soy sauce, 2 tablespoons of the lime juice, and the Sriracha and mix well. Set aside.
2.  Select the Sauté setting on the Instant Pot and heat the avocado oil, sesame oil, garlic, and ginger for 2 minutes, until the garlic is bubbling but not browned. Add the carrots, celery, and onion and sauté for about 3 minutes, until the onion begins to soften.
3.  Add the turkey and salt and sauté, using a wooden spoon or spatula to break up the meat as it cooks, for about 5 minutes, until cooked through and no streaks of pink remain. Add the water chestnuts and soy sauce mixture and stir to combine, working quickly so not too much steam escapes.
4.  Secure the lid and set the Pressure Release to Sealing. Press the Cancel button to reset the cooking program, then select the Manual setting and set the cooking time for 5 minutes at high pressure. (The pot will take about 10 minutes to come up to pressure before the cooking program begins.)
5.  When the cooking program ends, perform a quick pressure release by moving the Pressure Release to Venting, or let the pressure release naturally. Open the pot.
6.  In a small bowl, stir together the remaining 1 tablespoon lime juice and the cornstarch, add the mixture to the pot, and stir to combine. Press the Cancel button to reset the cooking program, then select the Sauté setting. Let the mixture come to a boil and thicken, stirring often, for about 2 minutes, then press the Cancel button to turn off the pot.
7.  Spoon the turkey mixture onto the lettuce leaves and sprinkle the cashews and cilantro on top. Serve right away, with additional Sriracha at the table.

**Per Serving**
calories: 306 | fat: 17g | protein: 26g | carbs: 12g | sugars: 2g | fiber: 4g | sodium: 303mg

# 7-Layer Dip



**Cashew Sour Cream:**
1 cup raw whole cashews, soaked in water to cover for 1 to 2 hours and then drained
½ cup avocado oil                                    ½ cup water
¼ cup fresh lemon juice                         2 tablespoons nutritional yeast
1 teaspoon fine sea salt
**Beans:**
½ cup dried black beans                        2 cups water
½ teaspoon fine sea salt                        ½ teaspoon chili powder
¼ teaspoon garlic powder

½ cup grape or cherry tomatoes, halved
1 avocado, diced
¼ cup chopped yellow onion                1 jalapeño chile, sliced
2 tablespoons chopped cilantro            6 ounces (170 g) baked corn tortilla chips
1 English cucumber, sliced                      2 carrots, sliced
6 celery stalks, cut into sticks

1.  To make the cashew sour cream: In a blender, combine the cashews, oil, water, lemon juice, nutritional yeast, and salt. Blend on high speed, stopping to scrape down the sides of the container as needed, for about 2 minutes, until very smooth. (The sour cream can be made in advance and stored in an airtight container in the refrigerator for up to 5 days.)
2.  To make the beans: Pour 1 cup water into the Instant Pot. In a 1½-quart stainless-steel bowl, combine the beans, the 2 cups water, and salt and stir to dissolve the salt. Place the bowl on a long-handled silicone steam rack, then, holding the handles of the steam rack, lower it into the Instant Pot. (If you don't have the long-handled rack, use the wire metal steam rack and a homemade sling)
3.  Secure the lid and set the Pressure Release to Sealing. Select the Bean/Chili or Manual setting and set the cooking time for 25 minutes at high pressure. (The pot will take about 10 minutes to come up to pressure before the cooking program begins.)
4.  When the cooking program ends, let the pressure release naturally for at least 20 minutes, then move the Pressure Release to Venting to release any remaining steam.
5.  Place a colander over a bowl. Open the pot and, wearing heat-resistant mitts, lift out the inner pot and drain the beans in the colander. Transfer the liquid captured in the bowl to a measuring cup, and pour the beans into the bowl. Add ¼ cup of the cooking liquid to the beans and, using a potato masher or fork, mash the beans to your desired consistency, adding more cooking liquid as needed. Stir in the chili powder and garlic powder.
6.  Using a rubber spatula, spread the black beans in an even layer in a clear-glass serving dish. Spread the cashew sour cream in an even layer on top of the beans. Add layers of the tomatoes, avocado, onion, jalapeño, and cilantro. (At this point, you can cover and refrigerate the assembled dip for up to 1 day.) Serve accompanied with the tortilla chips, cucumber, carrots, and celery on the side.

**Per Serving** (includes chips and vegetables for dipping)
calories: 259 | fat: 8g | protein: 8g | carbs: 41g | sugars: 3g | fiber: 8g | sodium: 811mg

# Lemon Artichokes

**Prep time: 5 minutes | Cook time: 5 to 15 minutes | Serves 4**

4 artichokes

2 tablespoons lemon juice

1 cup water

1 teaspoon salt

1. Wash and trim artichokes by cutting off the stems flush with the bottoms of the artichokes and by cutting ¾ to 1 inch off the tops. Stand upright in the bottom of the inner pot of the Instant Pot.
2. Pour water, lemon juice, and salt over artichokes.
3. Secure the lid and make sure the vent is set to sealing. On Manual, set the Instant Pot for 15 minutes for large artichokes, 10 minutes for medium artichokes, or 5 minutes for small artichokes.
4. When cook time is up, perform a quick release by releasing the pressure manually.

**Per Serving**
calories: 60 | fat: 0g | protein: 4g | carbs: 13g | sugars: 1g | fiber: 6g | sodium: 397mg

# Instant Popcorn

**Prep time: 1 minute | Cook time: 5 minutes | Serves 5**

2 tablespoons coconut oil

¼ cup margarine spread, melted, optional

½ cup popcorn kernels

Sea salt, to taste

1. Set the Instant Pot to Sauté.
2. Melt the coconut oil in the inner pot, then add the popcorn kernels and stir.
3. Press Adjust to bring the temperature up to high.
4. When the corn starts popping, secure the lid on the Instant Pot.
5. When you no longer hear popping, turn off the Instant Pot, remove the lid, and pour the popcorn into a bowl.
6. Top with the optional melted margarine and season the popcorn with sea salt to your liking.

**Per Serving**
calories: 161 | fat: 12g | protein: 1g | carbs: 13g | sugars: 0g | fiber: 3g | sodium: 89mg

# Blackberry Baked Brie

**Prep time: 5 minutes | Cook time: 15 minutes | Serves 5**

8 ounces (227 g) round Brie

¼ cup sugar-free blackberry preserves

1 cup water

2 teaspoons chopped fresh mint

1. Slice a grid pattern into the top of the rind of the Brie with a knife.
2. In a 7-inch round baking dish, place the Brie, then cover the baking dish securely with foil.
3. Insert the trivet into the inner pot of the Instant Pot; pour in the water.
4. Make a foil sling and arrange it on top of the trivet. Place the baking dish on top of the trivet and foil sling.
5. Secure the lid to the locked position and turn the vent to sealing.
6. Press Manual and set the Instant Pot for 15 minutes on high pressure.
7. When cooking time is up, turn off the Instant Pot and do a quick release of the pressure.
8. When the valve has dropped, remove the lid, then remove the baking dish.
9. Remove the top rind of the Brie and top with the preserves. Sprinkle with the fresh mint.

**Per Serving**
calories: 133 | fat: 10g | protein: 8g | carbs: 4g | sugars: 0g | fiber: 0g | sodium: 238mg

## Creamy Spinach Dip



8 ounces (227 g) low-fat cream cheese
½ cup finely chopped onion
5 cloves garlic, minced
¼ teaspoon black pepper
12 ounces (340 g) reduced-fat shredded Monterey Jack cheese
12 ounces (340 g) reduced-fat shredded Parmesan cheese

1 cup low-fat sour cream
½ cup no-sodium vegetable broth
½ teaspoon salt
10 ounces (283 g) frozen spinach

1. Add cream cheese, sour cream, onion, vegetable broth, garlic, salt, pepper, and spinach to the inner pot of the Instant Pot.
2. Secure lid, make sure vent is set to sealing, and set to the Bean/Chili setting on high pressure for 5 minutes.
3. When done, do a quick release.
4. Add the cheeses and mix well until creamy and well combined.

**Per Serving**
calories: 274 | fat: 18g | protein: 19g | carbs: 10g | sugars: 3g | fiber: 1g | sodium: 948mg

## Smoky Deviled Eggs

Prep time: 10 minutes | Cook time: 15 minutes | Serves 6

6 large eggs
1 teaspoon Dijon mustard
¾ teaspoon smoked paprika (sweet or hot), plus more for serving
1 tablespoon chopped fresh chives

3 tablespoons mayonnaise
1 teaspoon hot sauce (such as Tabasco or Crystal)

1. Pour 1 cup water into the Instant Pot and place the wire metal steam rack or an egg rack into the pot. Gently place the eggs on the rack, taking care not to crack the eggs as you add them.
2. Secure the lid and set the Pressure Release to Sealing. Select the Steam setting and set the cooking time for 5 minutes at high pressure. (The pot will take about 10 minutes to come up to pressure before the cooking program begins.)
3. While the eggs are cooking, prepare an ice bath.
4. When the cooking program ends, let the pressure release naturally for 5 minutes, then move the Pressure Release to Venting to release any remaining steam. Open the pot and transfer the eggs to the ice bath to cool for about 10 minutes.
5. Roll each egg around on the countertop to crack the entire shell and loosen the membrane, then, starting at the pointy end of the egg, peel off the shell. Slice the eggs in half lengthwise and transfer the yolks to a medium bowl. Arrange the egg white halves, hollow-side up, on a work surface.
6. Using a fork, mash the yolks thoroughly. Add the mayonnaise, mustard, hot sauce, and paprika and stir until the ingredients are evenly combined and the filling is smooth. Spoon or pipe the filling into the egg white halves. (At this point, you can store them in an airtight container in the refrigerator for up to 1 day.)
7. Sprinkle the deviled eggs with the chives and additional paprika before serving.

**Per Serving(2 halves)**
calories: 117 | fat: 10g | protein: 6g | carbs: 1g | sugars: 0g | fiber: 0g | sodium: 68mg

# Creamy Jalapeño Chicken Dip

**Prep time: 5 minutes | Cook time: 12 minutes | Serves 10**

1 pound (454 g) boneless chicken breast
3 jalapeños, seeded and sliced
8 ounces (227 g) reduced-fat shredded Cheddar cheese
¾ cup low-fat sour cream

8 ounces (227 g) low-fat cream cheese
½ cup water

1.  Place the chicken, cream cheese, jalapeños, and water in the inner pot of the Instant Pot.
2.  Secure the lid so it's locked and turn the vent to sealing.
3.  Press Manual and set the Instant Pot for 12 minutes on high pressure.
4.  When cooking time is up, turn off Instant Pot, do a quick release of the remaining pressure, then remove lid.
5.  Shred the chicken between 2 forks, either in the pot or on a cutting board, then place back in the inner pot.
6.  Stir in the shredded cheese and sour cream.

**Per Serving**
calories: 238 | fat: 13g | protein: 24g | carbs: 7g | sugars: 5g | fiber: 1g | sodium: 273mg

# Green Goddess White Bean Dip

**Prep time: 1 minute | Cook time: 45 minutes | Makes 3 cups**

1 cup dried navy, great Northern, or cannellini beans
4 cups water
3 tablespoons fresh lemon juice
¼ cup firmly packed fresh flat-leaf parsley leaves
1 bunch chives, chopped
Freshly ground black pepper, to taste

2 teaspoons fine sea salt
¼ cup extra-virgin olive oil, plus 1 tablespoon

Leaves from 2 tarragon sprigs

1.  Combine the beans, water, and 1 teaspoon of the salt in the Instant Pot and stir to dissolve the salt.
2.  Secure the lid and set the Pressure Release to Sealing. Select the Bean/Chili or Manual setting and set the cooking time for 30 minutes at high pressure if using navy or Great Northern beans or 40 minutes at high pressure if using cannellini beans. (The pot will take about 15 minutes to come up to pressure before the cooking program begins.)
3.  When the cooking program ends, let the pressure release naturally for 15 minutes, then move the Pressure Release to Venting to release any remaining steam. Open the pot and scoop out and reserve ½ cup of the cooking liquid. Wearing heat-resistant mitts, lift out the inner pot and drain the beans in a colander.
4.  In a food processor or blender, combine the beans, ½ cup cooking liquid, lemon juice, ¼ cup olive oil, ½ teaspoon parsley, chives, tarragon, remaining 1 teaspoon salt, and ½ teaspoon pepper. Process or blend on medium speed, stopping to scrape down the sides of the container as needed, for about 1 minute, until the mixture is smooth.
5.  Transfer the dip to a serving bowl. Drizzle with the remaining 1 tablespoon olive oil and sprinkle with a few grinds of pepper. The dip will keep in an airtight container in the refrigerator for up to 1 week. Serve at room temperature or chilled.

**Per Serving (¼ cup)**
calories: 70 | fat: 5g | protein: 3g | carbs: 8g | sugars: 1g | fiber: 4g | sodium: 782mg

## Porcupine Meatballs

**Prep time: 20 minutes | Cook time: 15 minutes | Serves 8**

1 pound (454 g) ground sirloin or turkey
1 egg
1 or 2 cloves garlic, minced
¼ teaspoon dried basil and/or oregano, optional
1 (10¾-ounce / 305-g) can reduced-fat condensed tomato soup
½ soup can of water

½ cup raw brown rice, parboiled
¼ cup finely minced onion

1. Mix all ingredients, except tomato soup and water, in a bowl to combine well.
2. Form into balls about 1½-inch in diameter.
3. Mix tomato soup and water in the inner pot of the Instant Pot, then add the meatballs.
4. Secure the lid and make sure the vent is turned to sealing.
5. Press the Meat/Stew button and set for 15 minutes on high pressure.
6. Allow the pressure to release naturally after cook time is up.

**Per Serving**
calories: 141 | fat: 2g | protein: 16g | carbs: 14g | sugars: 3g | fiber: 1g | sodium: 176mg

## Buffalo Chicken Dip

**Prep time: 15 minutes | Cook time: 15 minutes | Serves 26**

2 large frozen boneless skinless chicken breasts
¾ cup Frank's RedHot sauce
½ cup sodium-free chicken broth
1 cup light ranch dressing
2 (8-ounce / 227-g) packages fat-free cream cheese, softened
1½ cups reduced-fat shredded Cheddar Jack cheese

1. Place the frozen chicken, hot sauce, and chicken broth into the inner pot of the Instant Pot. Secure the lid and make sure the vent is set to sealing.
2. Set the Instant Pot for 10 minutes on Manual. When cooking time is over, let the pressure release naturally for 10 minutes and then perform a quick release.
3. Remove the lid and press Cancel. Then choose Sauté low.
4. Stir in the ranch dressing, cream cheese, and Cheddar Jack cheese. Cook, stirring until well blended and warm.

**Per Serving**
calories: 84 | fat: 3g | protein: 10g | carbs: 2g | sugars: 1g | fiber: 1g | sodium: 443mg

# Artichoke Spinach Dip

**Prep time: 5 minutes | Cook time: 15 minutes | Makes 4½ cups**

1 tablespoon extra-virgin olive oil

1 large yellow onion, diced

½ teaspoon freshly ground black pepper

1½ teaspoons Italian seasoning

4 garlic cloves, minced

½ teaspoon fine sea salt

½ cup low-sodium vegetable broth

1 (12-ounce / 340-g) bag frozen artichoke hearts, thawed according to package directions, drained, and chopped

1 (1-pound / 454-g) bag frozen chopped spinach, thawed according to package directions and squeezed of excess moisture

1 cup raw whole cashews, soaked in water to cover for 1 to 2 hours and then drained

¼ cup fresh lemon juice

¼ cup unsweetened soy milk or almond milk

2 tablespoons nutritional yeast

1. Select the Sauté setting on the Instant Pot and heat the oil and garlic for 3 minutes, until the garlic is bubbling but not browned. Add the onion, salt, and pepper and sauté for 4 minutes, until the onion begins to soften. Stir in the broth, Italian seasoning, artichoke hearts, and spinach, using a wooden spoon or spatula to nudge any browned bits from the bottom of the pot and working quickly so not too much liquid evaporates.
2. Secure the lid and set the Pressure Release to Sealing. Press the Cancel button to reset the cooking program, then select the Manual setting and set the cooking time for 1 minute at high pressure. (The pot will take about 5 minutes to come up to pressure before the cooking program begins.)
3. While the vegetables are cooking, in a widemouthed pint jar, combine the cashews, lemon juice, soy milk, and nutritional yeast. Using an immersion blender, blend the mixture for about 2 minutes, until smooth.
4. When the cooking program ends, perform a quick release by moving the Pressure Release to Venting, or let the pressure release naturally. Open the pot and, wearing heat-resistant mitts, lift the inner pot out of the housing. Add the cashew mixture and stir until well combined.
5. Transfer the dip to a serving bowl and serve warm.

**Per Serving (¼ cup)**

calories: 127 | fat: 7g | protein: 6g | carbs: 10g | sugars: 2g | fiber: 3g | sodium: 392mg

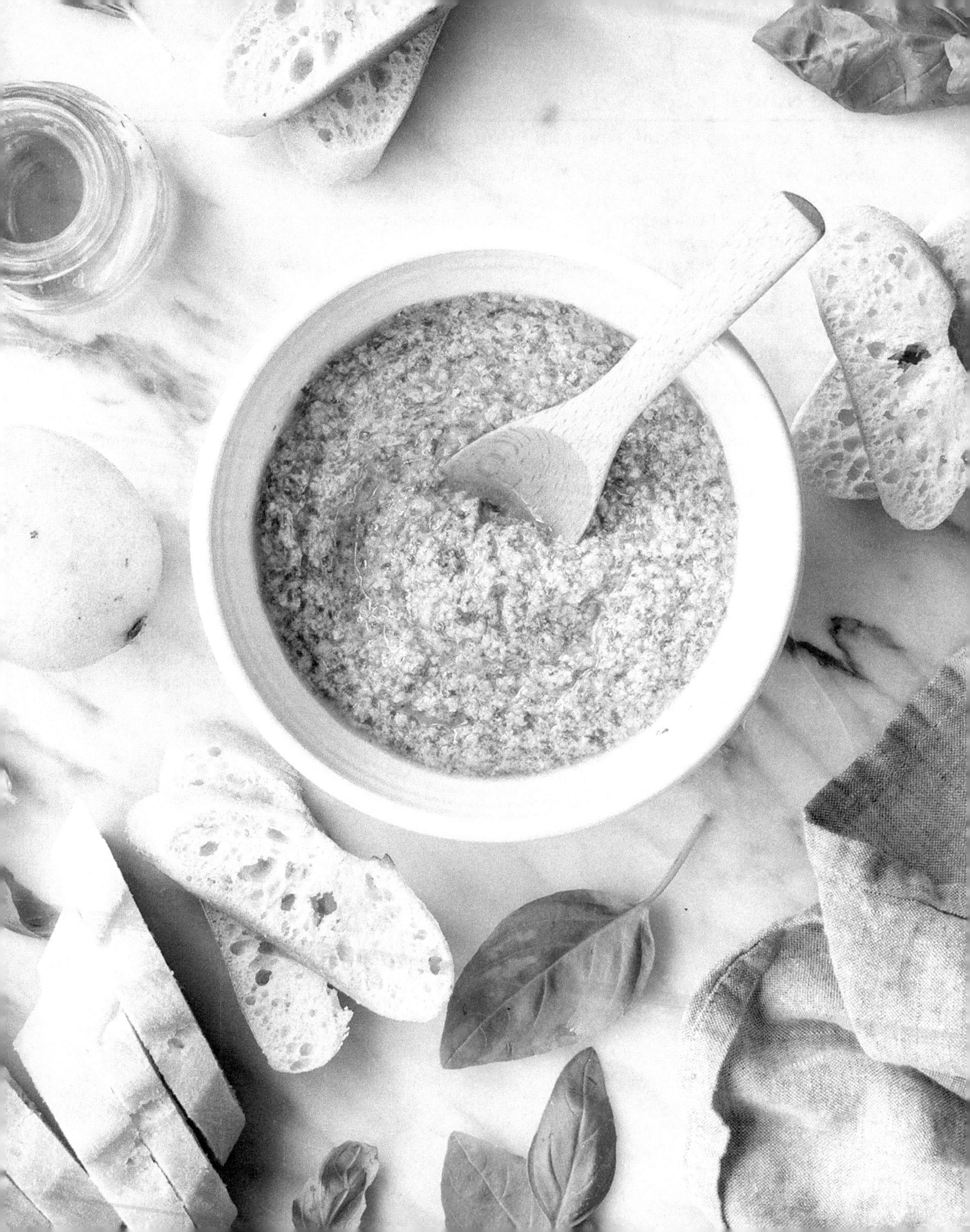

# Chapter 5 Soups and Stews

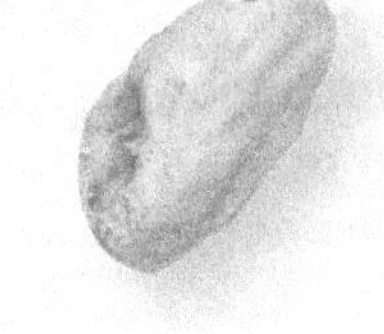


39   Chicken Rice Soup   40

40   Creamy Sweet Potato Soup   40

41   Chicken Noodle Soup   41

42   Unstuffed Cabbage Soup   41

43   Buttercup Squash Soup   42

44   Turkey Barley Vegetable Soup   42

45   French Market Soup   43

46   Southwestern Bean Soup with Corn Dumplings   43

47   Beef Stew   44

48   Alpine Pork and Apple Stew   45

49   Brown Lentil Soup   46

50   Split Pea Soup   46

51   French Onion Soup   47

52   Instantly Good Beef Stew   47

53   Ground Turkey Stew   48

54   Hearty Hamburger and Lentil Stew   48

55   Favorite Chili   49

56   Chicken Vegetable Soup   50

57   Tuscan Beef Stew   50

58   Easy Southern Brunswick Stew   51

59   Three-Bean Chili   51

60   Pork Chili   52

61   Vegetarian Chili   52

62   Turkey and Pinto Chili   53


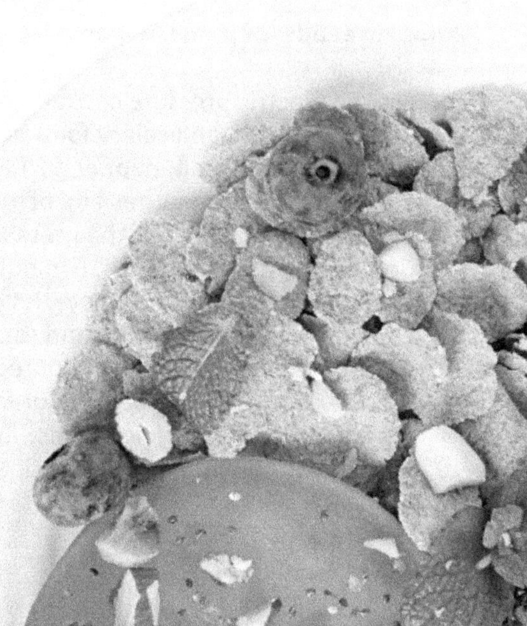

# Chicken Rice Soup



**Prep time: 10 minutes | Cook time: 10 minutes | Serves 8**

1 teaspoon vegetable oil

1 medium onion, chopped

½ cup long-grain rice, uncooked

1 pound (454 g) boneless skinless chicken breasts, cut into ¾-inch cubes

5¼ cups fat-free, low-sodium chicken broth

2 teaspoons dried thyme leaves

2 ribs celery, chopped into ½-inch-thick pieces

1 cup wild rice, uncooked

¼ teaspoon red pepper flakes

1. Using the Sauté function on the Instant Pot, heat the teaspoon of vegetable oil. Sauté the celery and onion until the onions are slightly translucent (3 to 5 minutes). Once cooked, press Cancel.
2. Add the remaining ingredients to the inner pot.
3. Secure the lid and make sure the vent is set to sealing. Using the Manual function, set the time to 10 minutes.
4. When cook time is over, let the pressure release naturally for 10 minutes, then perform a quick release.

**Per Serving**
calories: 160 | fat: 2g | protein: 16g | carbs: 18g | sugars: 2g | fiber: 1g | sodium: 375mg

# Creamy Sweet Potato Soup

**Prep time: 15 minutes | Cook time: 10 minutes | Serves 6**

2 tablespoons avocado oil

2 celery stalks, chopped

1 teaspoon kosher salt

1 teaspoon ground turmeric

2 pounds (907 g) sweet potatoes, peeled and cut into 1-inch cubes

3 cups vegetable broth or chicken bone broth

Plain Greek yogurt, to garnish (optional)

Pumpkin seeds (pepitas), to garnish (optional)

1 small onion, chopped

2 teaspoons minced garlic

½ teaspoon freshly ground black pepper

½ teaspoon ground cinnamon

Chopped fresh parsley, to garnish (optional)

1. Set the electric pressure cooker to the Sauté setting. When the pot is hot, pour in the avocado oil.
2. Sauté the onion and celery for 3 to 5 minutes or until the vegetables begin to soften.
3. Stir in the garlic, salt, pepper, turmeric, and cinnamon. Hit Cancel.
4. Stir in the sweet potatoes and broth.
5. Close and lock the lid of the pressure cooker. Set the valve to sealing.
6. Cook on high pressure for 10 minutes.
7. When the cooking is complete, hit Cancel and allow the pressure to release naturally.
8. Once the pin drops, unlock and remove the lid.
9. Use an immersion blender to purée the soup right in the pot. If you don't have an immersion blender, transfer the soup to a blender or food processor and purée. (Follow the instructions that came with your machine for blending hot foods.)
10. Spoon into bowls and serve topped with Greek yogurt, parsley, and/or pumpkin seeds (if using).

**Per Serving (1 cup)**
calories: 193 | fat: 5g | protein: 3g | carbs: 36g | sugars: 8g | fiber: 6g | sodium: 302mg

# Chicken Noodle Soup



**Prep time: 15 minutes | Cook time: 20 minutes | Serves 12**

2 tablespoons avocado oil

3 celery stalks, chopped

¼ teaspoon freshly ground black pepper

5 large carrots, peeled and cut into ¼-inch-thick rounds

3 pounds (1.4 kg) bone-in chicken breasts (about 3)

4 cups water

6 ounces (170 g) whole grain wide egg noodles

1 medium onion, chopped

1 teaspoon kosher salt

2 teaspoons minced garlic

4 cups low-sodium store-bought chicken broth

2 tablespoons soy sauce

1. Set the electric pressure cooker to the Sauté setting. When the pot is hot, pour in the avocado oil.
2. Sauté the onion, celery, salt, and pepper for 3 to 5 minutes or until the vegetables begin to soften.
3. Add the garlic and carrots, and stir to mix well. Hit Cancel.
4. Add the chicken to the pot, meat-side down. Add the broth, water, and soy sauce. Close and lock the lid of the pressure cooker. Set the valve to sealing.
5. Cook on high pressure for 20 minutes.
6. When the cooking is complete, hit Cancel and quick release the pressure. Unlock and remove the lid.
7. Using tongs, remove the chicken breasts to a cutting board. Hit Sauté/More and bring the soup to a boil.
8. Add the noodles and cook for 4 to 5 minutes or until the noodles are al dente.
9. While the noodles are cooking, use two forks to shred the chicken. Add the meat back to the pot and save the bones to make more bone broth.
10. Season with additional pepper, if desired, and serve.

**Per Serving (1 cup)**
calories: 330 | fat: 15g | protein: 32g | carbs: 17g | sugars: 3g | fiber: 4g | sodium: 451mg

# Unstuffed Cabbage Soup

**Prep time: 15 minutes | Cook time: 20 minutes | Serves 5**

2 tablespoons coconut oil

1 medium onion, diced

1 small head cabbage, chopped, cored, cut into roughly 2-inch pieces

1 (6-ounce / 170-g) can low-sodium tomato paste

1 (32-ounce / 907-g) can low-sodium diced tomatoes, with liquid

2 cups low-sodium beef broth

¾ cup brown rice

½ teaspoon black pepper

1 teaspoon parsley

1 pound (454 g) ground sirloin or turkey

2 cloves garlic, minced

1½ cups water

1 to 2 teaspoons salt

1 teaspoon oregano

1. Melt coconut oil in the inner pot of the Instant Pot using Sauté function. Add ground meat. Stir frequently until meat loses color, about 2 minutes.
2. Add onion and garlic and continue to sauté for 2 more minutes, stirring frequently.
3. Add chopped cabbage.
4. On top of cabbage layer tomato paste, tomatoes with liquid, beef broth, water, rice, and spices.
5. Secure the lid and set vent to sealing. Using Manual setting, select 20 minutes.
6. When time is up, let the pressure release naturally for 10 minutes, then do a quick release.

**Per Serving**
calories: 282 | fat: 6g | protein: 23g | carbs: 34g | sugars: 6g | fiber: 3g | sodium: 898mg

# Buttercup Squash Soup

**Prep time: 15 minutes | Cook time: 10 minutes | Serves 6**

2 tablespoons extra-virgin olive oil

1 medium onion, chopped

4 to 5 cups vegetable broth or chicken bone broth

1½ pounds (680 g) buttercup squash, peeled, seeded, and cut into 1-inch chunks

½ teaspoon kosher salt

¼ teaspoon ground white pepper

Whole nutmeg, for grating

1. Set the electric pressure cooker to the Sauté setting. When the pot is hot, pour in the olive oil.
2. Add the onion and sauté for 3 to 5 minutes, until it begins to soften. Hit Cancel.
3. Add the broth, squash, salt, and pepper to the pot and stir. (If you want a thicker soup, use 4 cups of broth. If you want a thinner, drinkable soup, use 5 cups.)
4. Close and lock the lid of the pressure cooker. Set the valve to sealing.
5. Cook on high pressure for 10 minutes.
6. When the cooking is complete, hit Cancel and allow the pressure to release naturally.
7. Once the pin drops, unlock and remove the lid.
8. Use an immersion blender to purée the soup right in the pot. If you don't have an immersion blender, transfer the soup to a blender or food processor and purée. (Follow the instructions that came with your machine for blending hot foods.)
9. Pour the soup into serving bowls and grate nutmeg on top.

**Per Serving (1⅓ cups)**
calories: 110 | fat: 5g | protein: 1g | carbs: 18g | sugars: 4g | fiber: 4g | sodium: 166mg

# Turkey Barley Vegetable Soup

**Prep time: 5 minutes | Cook time: 20 minutes | Serves 8**

2 tablespoons avocado oil

1 pound (454 g) ground turkey

4 cups low-sodium store-bought chicken broth or water

1 (28-ounce / 794-g) carton or can diced tomatoes    2 tablespoons tomato paste

1 (15-ounce / 425-g) package frozen chopped carrots (about 2½ cups)

1 (15-ounce / 425-g) package frozen peppers and onions (about 2½ cups)

⅓ cup dry barley

1 teaspoon kosher salt

¼ teaspoon freshly ground black pepper

2 bay leaves

1. Set the electric pressure cooker to the Sauté/More setting. When the pot is hot, pour in the avocado oil.
2. Add the turkey to the pot and sauté, stirring frequently to break up the meat, for about 7 minutes or until the turkey is no longer pink. Hit Cancel.
3. Add the broth, tomatoes and their juices, and tomato paste. Stir in the carrots, peppers and onions, barley, salt, pepper, and bay leaves.
4. Close and lock the lid of the pressure cooker. Set the valve to sealing.
5. Cook on high pressure for 20 minutes.
6. When the cooking is complete, hit Cancel and allow the pressure to release naturally for 10 minutes, then quick release any remaining pressure.
7. Once the pin drops, unlock and remove the lid. Discard the bay leaves.
8. Spoon into bowls and serve.

**Per Serving (1¼ cups)**
calories: 253 | fat: 12g | protein: 19g | carbs: 21g | sugars: 7g | fiber: 7g | sodium: 560mg

# French Market Soup



**Prep time: 20 minutes | Cook time: 1 hour | Serves 8**

2 cups mixed dry beans, washed with stones removed   7 cups water
1 ham hock, all visible fat removed                 1 teaspoon salt
¼ teaspoon pepper                                   1 (16-ounce / 454-g) can low-sodium tomatoes
1 large onion, chopped                              1 garlic clove, minced
1 chile, chopped, or 1 teaspoon chili powder        ¼ cup lemon juice

1. Combine all ingredients in the inner pot of the Instant Pot.
2. Secure the lid and make sure vent is set to sealing. Using Manual, set the Instant Pot to cook for 60 minutes.
3. When cooking time is over, let the pressure release naturally. When the Instant Pot is ready, unlock the lid, then remove the bone and any hard or fatty pieces. Pull the meat off the bone and chop into small pieces. Add the ham back into the Instant Pot.

**Per Serving**
calories: 191 | fat: 4g | protein: 12g | carbs: 29g | sugars: 5g | fiber: 7g | sodium: 488mg

# Southwestern Bean Soup with Corn Dumplings

**Prep time: 50 minutes | Cook time: 4 to 12 hours | Serves 8**

1 (15½-ounce / 439-g) can red kidney beans, rinsed and drained
1 (15½-ounce / 439-g) can black beans, pinto beans, or great northern beans, rinsed and drained
3 cups water
1 (14½-ounce / 411-g) can Mexican-style stewed tomatoes
1 (10-ounce / 283-g) package frozen whole-kernel corn, thawed
1 cup sliced carrots                                1 cup chopped onions
1 (4-ounce / 113-g) can chopped green chilies
3 teaspoons sodium-free instant bouillon powder (any flavor)
1 to 2 teaspoons chili powder                       2 cloves garlic, minced
Sauce:
⅓ cup flour                                         ¼ cup yellow cornmeal
1 teaspoon baking powder                            Dash of pepper
1 egg white, beaten                                 2 tablespoons milk
1 tablespoon oil

1. Combine the 11 soup ingredients in inner pot of the Instant Pot.
2. Secure the lid and cook on the low Slow Cook setting for 10 to 12 hours or high for 4 to 5 hours.
3. Make dumplings by mixing together flour, cornmeal, baking powder, and pepper.
4. Combine egg white, milk, and oil. Add to flour mixture. Stir with fork until just combined.
5. At the end of the soup's cooking time, turn the Instant Pot to Slow Cook function high if you don't already have it there. Remove the lid and drop dumpling mixture by rounded teaspoonfuls to make 8 mounds atop the soup.
6. Secure the lid once more and cook for an additional 30 minutes.

**Per Serving**
calories: 197 | fat: 1g | protein: 9g | carbs: 39g | sugars: 6g | fiber: 8g | sodium: 367mg

# Beef Stew



2 pounds (907 g) chuck steak, 1½-inch thickness
Salt, to taste
1 tablespoon Worcestershire sauce
3 tablespoons low-sodium tomato paste
12 white mushrooms, thinly sliced
Olive oil, optional
2 celery stalks, cut into 1½-inch chunks
¼ cup apple juice
¼ teaspoon dried thyme
1 tablespoon flour

Black pepper, to taste
1 tablespoon low-sodium soy sauce
1½ cups low-sodium chicken stock
2 small onions, thinly sliced
3 cloves garlic, crushed and minced
2 carrots, cut into 1½-inch chunks
2 bay leaves
3 to 4 small Yukon Gold potatoes, quartered
½ cup frozen peas

1. Heat up your Instant Pot by pressing the Sauté button and click the adjust button to go to Sauté More function. Wait until the indicator says "hot".
2. Season one side of the chuck steak generously with salt and ground black pepper. Add olive oil into the inner pot. Be sure to coat the oil over whole bottom of the pot.
3. Carefully place the seasoned side of chuck steak in the inner pot. Generously season the other side with salt and ground black pepper. Brown for 6 to 8 minutes on each side without constantly flipping the steak. Remove and set aside in a large mixing bowl.
4. While the chuck steak is browning, mix together the Worcestershire sauce, soy sauce, and tomato paste with the chicken stock.
5. Add sliced mushrooms into the Instant Pot. Sauté until all moisture from the mushrooms has evaporated and the edges are slightly crisped and browned, about 6 minutes. Taste and season with salt and ground black pepper if necessary. Remove and set aside.
6. Add olive oil into Instant Pot if necessary. Add onions and sauté until softened and slightly browned. Add garlic and stir for roughly 30 seconds until fragrant.
7. Add all celery and carrots and sauté until slightly browned. Season with salt and freshly ground black pepper if necessary.
8. Pour in apple juice and completely deglaze bottom of the pot by scrubbing the flavorful brown bits with a wooden spoon.
9. Add 2 bay leaves, dried thyme, quartered potatoes, and chicken stock mixture in the pot. Mix well. Close and secure lid and pressure cook on Manual at high pressure for 4 minutes. When time is up, quick release the pressure. Open the lid.
10. While the vegetables are pressure cooking, cut the chuck steak into 1-inch cubes on a large chopping board.
11. Place all chuck stew meat and the flavorful meat juice back in the large mixing bowl. Add flour in mixing bowl and mix well with the stew meat.
12. Remove half of the carrots, celery, and potatoes from pressure cooker and set aside. Place beef stew meat and all its juice in the inner pot. Partially submerge the beef stew meat in the liquid without stirring, as you don't want too much flour in the liquid at this point.
13. Close and secure the lid and pressure cook on Manual at high pressure for 32 minutes. When time is up, turn off the Instant Pot and quick release any remaining pressure.
14. On medium heat by pressing the Sauté button, break down the mushy potatoes and carrots with a wooden spoon. Stir to thicken the stew.

15.    Add frozen peas, sautéed mushrooms, and the set-aside carrots, celery, and potatoes in the pot.
       Taste and season with salt and ground black pepper if necessary.
16.    Serve with mashed potatoes, pasta, or your favorite starch. Enjoy!

**Per Serving**
calories: 445 | fat: 25g | protein: 33g | carbs: 23g | sugars: 6g | fiber: 4g | sodium: 363mg

## Alpine Pork and Apple Stew

**Prep time: 10 minutes | Cook time: 55 minutes | Serves 6**

**2 pounds (907 g) pork stew meat or boneless pork loin roast, cut into 1½-inch pieces**
**1½ teaspoons fine sea salt**
**½ teaspoon freshly ground black pepper**
**2 tablespoons cold-pressed avocado oil**
**1 large yellow onion, chopped**
**3 garlic cloves, minced**
**1 cup dry hard cider or dry white wine**
**1 teaspoon dried thyme**
**1 teaspoon dried sage**
**½ teaspoon dried rosemary**
**¼ teaspoon cayenne pepper**
**1 pound (454 g) carrots, cut into bite-size pieces**
**2 large Granny Smith or other tart baking apples, each cut into 12 wedges**

1.    Sprinkle the pork all over with the salt and black pepper.
2.    Select the Sauté setting on the Instant Pot and heat the oil for 3 minutes, until shimmering. Using tongs, add
      half of the pork in a single layer and sear for about 4 minutes, until lightly browned on one side. Transfer the
      pork to a plate. Repeat with the remaining pork.
3.    Add the onion and garlic to the pot and sauté for 3 minutes, until the onion begins to soften. Add the cider
      and use a wooden spoon or spatula to nudge any browned bits from the bottom of the pot. Stir in the thyme,
      sage, rosemary, and cayenne and then return the pork to the pot.
4.    Press the Cancel button to reset the cooking program, then select the Meat/Stew or Manual setting and set
      the cooking time for 20 minutes at high pressure. (The pot will take about 5 minutes to come up to pressure
      before the cooking program begins.)
5.    When the cooking program ends, perform a quick pressure release by moving the Pressure Release to
      Venting, or let the pressure release naturally. Open the pot and layer the carrots and apples on top of the
      pork.
6.    Secure the lid and set the Pressure Release to Sealing. Press the Cancel button to reset the cooking program,
      then select the Manual setting and set the cooking time for 2 minutes at low pressure. (The pot will take
      about 10 minutes to come up to pressure before the cooking program begins.)
7.    When the cooking program ends, perform a quick pressure release by moving the Pressure Release to
      Venting. Open the pot and stir the stew to mix all of the ingredients.
8.    Spoon the stew into bowls and serve hot.

**Per Serving**
calories: 343 | fat: 14g | protein: 28g | carbs: 22g | sugars: 10g | fiber: 5g | sodium: 902mg

# Brown Lentil Soup

**Prep time: 15 minutes | Cook time: 20 minutes | Serves 4**

1 medium onion, chopped
1 medium carrot, diced
1 small bay leaf
5 cups low-sodium chicken broth
½ teaspoon lemon juice

1 tablespoon olive oil
2 cloves garlic, minced
1 pound (454 g) brown lentils
¼ teaspoon ground black pepper

1. Using the Sauté function, sauté the chopped onion in oil in the inner pot of the Instant Pot about 2 minutes, or until it starts to soften.
2. Add diced carrot and sauté 3 minutes more until it begins to soften. Stir frequently or it will stick.
3. Add garlic and sauté 1 more minute.
4. Add bay leaf, lentils, and broth to pot.
5. Secure the lid and make sure vent is at sealing. Using Manual setting, select 14 minutes and cook on high pressure.
6. When cooking time is up, do a quick release of the pressure.
7. Discard bay leaf.
8. Stir in pepper and lemon juice, then adjust seasonings to taste.

**Per Serving**
calories: 151 | fat: 4g | protein: 10g | carbs: 5g | sugars: 3g | fiber: 1g | sodium: 79mg

# Split Pea Soup

**Prep time: 20 minutes | Cook time: 15 minutes | Serves 4**

4 cups low-sodium chicken broth
4 ounces (113 g) ham, diced (about ⅓ cup)
2 tablespoons margarine
2 carrots
3 cloves garlic
Salt and pepper, to taste

4 sprigs thyme

2 stalks celery
1 large leek
1½ cups dried green split peas (about 12 ounces / 340 g)

1. Pour the broth into the inner pot of the Instant Pot and set to Sauté. Add the thyme, ham, and margarine.
2. While the broth heats, chop the celery and cut the carrots into ½-inch-thick rounds. Halve the leek lengthwise and thinly slice and chop the garlic. Add the vegetables to the pot as you cut them. Rinse the split peas in a colander, discarding any stones, then add to the pot.
3. Secure the lid, making sure the steam valve is in the sealing position. Set the cooker to Manual at high pressure for 15 minutes. When the time is up, carefully turn the steam valve to the venting position to release the pressure manually.
4. Turn off the Instant Pot. Remove the lid and stir the soup; discard the thyme sprigs.
5. Thin the soup with up to one cup water if needed (the soup will continue to thicken as it cools). Season with salt and pepper.

**Per Serving**
calories: 200 | fat: 9g | protein: 12g | carbs: 20g | sugars: 3g | fiber: 2g | sodium: 450mg

# French Onion Soup

**Prep time: 10 minutes | Cook time: 20 minutes | Serves 10**

½ cup light, soft tub margarine

8 to 10 large onions, sliced

3 (14-ounce / 397-g) cans 98% fat-free, lower-sodium beef broth

2½ cups water

3 teaspoons sodium-free chicken bouillon powder

1½ teaspoons Worcestershire sauce

3 bay leaves

10 (1-ounce / 28-g) slices French bread, toasted

1. Turn the Instant Pot to the Sauté function and add in the margarine and onions. Cook about 5 minutes, or until the onions are slightly soft. Press Cancel.
2. Add the beef broth, water, bouillon powder, Worcestershire sauce, and bay leaves and stir.
3. Secure the lid and make sure vent is set to sealing. Cook on Manual mode for 20 minutes.
4. Let the pressure release naturally for 15 minutes, then do a quick release. Open the lid and discard bay leaves.
5. Ladle into bowls. Top each with a slice of bread and some cheese if you desire.

**Per Serving**

calories: 178 | fat: 4g | protein: 6g | carbs: 31g | sugars: 10g | fiber: 4g | sodium: 476mg

# Instantly Good Beef Stew

**Prep time: 20 minutes | Cook time: 35 minutes | Serves 6**

3 tablespoons olive oil, divided

2 pounds (907 g) stewing beef, cubed

2 cloves garlic, minced

1 large onion, chopped

3 ribs celery, sliced

3 large potatoes, cubed

2 to 3 carrots, sliced

8 ounces (227 g) no-salt-added tomato sauce

10 ounces (283 g) low-sodium beef broth

2 teaspoons Worcestershire sauce

¼ teaspoon pepper

1 bay leaf

1. Set the Instant Pot to the Sauté function, then add in 1 tablespoon of the oil. Add in ⅓ of the beef cubes and brown and sear all sides. Repeat this process twice more with the remaining oil and beef cubes. Set the beef aside.
2. Place the garlic, onion, and celery into the pot and sauté for a few minutes. Press Cancel.
3. Add the beef back in as well as all of the remaining ingredients.
4. Secure the lid and make sure the vent is set to sealing. Choose Manual for 35 minutes.
5. When cook time is up, let the pressure release naturally for 15 minutes, then release any remaining pressure manually.
6. Remove the lid, remove the bay leaf, then serve.

**Per Serving**

calories: 401 | fat: 20g | protein: 35g | carbs: 19g | sugars: 5g | fiber: 3g | sodium: 157mg

# Ground Turkey Stew



1 tablespoon olive oil
1 pound (454 g) ground turkey
1 teaspoon chili powder
2 teaspoons coriander
½ teaspoon salt
1 red pepper, chopped
1½ cups reduced-sodium tomato sauce
1 cup water
1 (15-ounce / 425-g) can reduced-salt black beans

1 onion, chopped
½ teaspoon garlic powder
¾ teaspoon cumin
1 teaspoon dried oregano
1 green pepper, chopped
1 tomato, chopped
1 tablespoon low-sodium soy sauce
2 handfuls cilantro, chopped

1. Press the Sauté function on the control panel of the Instant Pot.
2. Add the olive oil to the inner pot and let it get hot. Add onion and sauté for a few minutes, or until light golden.
3. Add ground turkey. Break the ground meat using a wooden spoon to avoid formation of lumps. Sauté for a few minutes, until the pink color has faded.
4. Add garlic powder, chili powder, cumin, coriander, dried oregano, and salt. Combine well. Add green pepper, red pepper, and chopped tomato. Combine well.
5. Add tomato sauce, soy sauce, and water; combine well.
6. Close and secure the lid. Click on the Cancel key to cancel the Sauté mode. Make sure the pressure release valve on the lid is in the sealing position.
7. Click on Manual function first and then select high pressure. Click the "+" button and set the time to 15 minutes.
8. You can either have the steam release naturally (it will take around 20 minutes) or, after 10 minutes, turn the pressure release valve on the lid to venting and release steam. Be careful as the steam is very hot. After the pressure has released completely, open the lid.
9. If the stew is watery, turn on the Sauté function and let it cook for a few more minutes with the lid off.
10. Add cilantro and can of black beans, combine well, and let cook for a few minutes.

**Per Serving**
calories: 209 | fat: 3g | protein: 24g | carbs: 21g | sugars: 8g | fiber: 6g | sodium: 609mg

# Hearty Hamburger and Lentil Stew



2 tablespoons cold-pressed avocado oil
1 large yellow onion, diced
2 celery stalks, diced
2 pounds (907 g) 95 percent lean ground beef
½ cup small green lentils
2 cups low-sodium roasted beef bone broth or vegetable broth
1 tablespoon Italian seasoning
1½ teaspoons fine sea salt
1 cup frozen green peas

2 garlic cloves, chopped
2 carrots, diced

1 tablespoon paprika
1 extra-large russet potato, diced
1 cup frozen corn

1 (14½-ounce / 411-g) can no-salt petite diced tomatoes and their liquid
¼ cup tomato paste

1. Select the Sauté setting on the Instant Pot and heat the oil and garlic for 3 minutes, until the garlic is bubbling but not browned. Add the onion, carrots, and celery and sauté for 5 minutes, until the onion begins to soften. Add the beef and sauté, using a wooden spoon or spatula to break up the meat as it cooks, for 6 minutes, until cooked through and no streaks of pink remain.
2. Stir in the lentils, broth, Italian seasoning, paprika, and salt. Add the potato, peas, corn, and tomatoes and their liquid in layers on top of the lentils and beef, then add the tomato paste in a dollop on top. Do not stir in the vegetables and tomato paste.
3. Secure the lid and set the Pressure Release to Sealing. Press the Cancel button to reset the cooking program, then select the Manual setting and set the cooking time for 20 minutes at high pressure. (The pot will take about 20 minutes to come up to pressure before the cooking program begins.)
4. When the cooking program ends, let the pressure release naturally for at least 15 minutes, then move the Pressure Release to Venting to release any remaining steam. Open the pot and stir the stew to mix all of the ingredients.
5. Ladle the stew into bowls and serve hot.

**Per Serving**
calories: 334 | fat: 8g | protein: 34g | carbs: 30g | sugars: 6g | fiber: 7g | sodium: 902mg

## Favorite Chili

**Prep time: 10 minutes | Cook time: 35 minutes | Serves 5**

1 pound (454 g) extra-lean ground beef
½ teaspoon black pepper
1 small onion, chopped
1 green pepper, chopped
½ teaspoon cumin
1 (16-ounce / 454-g) can chili beans

1 teaspoon salt
1 tablespoon olive oil
2 cloves garlic, minced
2 tablespoons chili powder
1 cup water
1 (15-ounce / 425-g) can low-sodium crushed tomatoes

1. Press Sauté button and adjust once to Sauté More function. Wait until indicator says "hot".
2. Season the ground beef with salt and black pepper.
3. Add the olive oil into the inner pot. Coat the whole bottom of the pot with the oil.
4. Add ground beef into the inner pot. The ground beef will start to release moisture. Allow the ground beef to brown and crisp slightly, stirring occasionally to break it up. Taste and adjust the seasoning with more salt and ground black pepper.
5. Add diced onion, minced garlic, chopped pepper, chili powder, and cumin. Sauté for about 5 minutes, until the spices start to release their fragrance. Stir frequently.
6. Add water and 1 can of chili beans, not drained. Mix well. Pour in 1 can of crushed tomatoes.
7. Close and secure lid, making sure vent is set to sealing, and pressure cook on Manual at high pressure for 10 minutes.
8. Let the pressure release naturally when cooking time is up. Open the lid carefully.

**Per Serving**
calories: 213 | fat: 10g | protein: 18g | carbs: 11g | sugars: 4g | fiber: 4g | sodium: 385mg

# Chicken Vegetable Soup



1 to 2 raw chicken breasts, cubed
4 cloves garlic, minced
1 large carrot, peeled and cubed
½ cup frozen corn
¼ cup frozen peas
¼ cup frozen lima beans
1 cup frozen green beans (bite-sized)
¼ to ½ cup chopped savoy cabbage
1 (14½-ounce / 411-g) can low-sodium petite diced tomatoes
3 cups low-sodium chicken bone broth
½ teaspoon black pepper
1 teaspoon garlic powder
¼ cup chopped fresh parsley
¼ to ½ teaspoon red pepper flakes

½ medium onion, chopped
½ sweet potato, small cubes
4 stalks celery, chopped, leaves included

1. Add all of the ingredients, in the order listed, to the inner pot of the Instant Pot.
2. Lock the lid in place, set the vent to sealing, press Manual, and cook at high pressure for 4 minutes.
3. Release the pressure manually as soon as cooking time is finished.

**Per Serving**
calories: 176 | fat: 3g | protein: 21g | carbs: 18g | sugars: 7g | fiber: 4g | sodium: 169mg

# Tuscan Beef Stew



1 (10½-ounce / 298-g) can tomato soup
1 (10½-ounce / 298-g) can fat-free, low-sodium beef broth
½ cup water
1 teaspoon Italian seasoning
½ teaspoon garlic powder
1 (14½-ounce / 411-g) can Italian diced tomatoes
¾ pound (340 g) carrot chunks (1-inch pieces)
2 pounds (907 g) stewing beef, cut into 1-inch cubes
2 (15½-ounce / 439-g) cans cannellini beans, rinsed and drained

1. Mix all ingredients except beans in the inner pot of the Instant Pot.
2. Secure the lid and set the Instant Pot to the Slow Cook mode on high for 4 to 5 hours, or on low 8 to 9 hours, or until vegetables and beef are tender.
3. Remove the lid, add in the beans, and cook on Slow Cook mode once more, high for 10 more minutes.

**Per Serving**
calories: 260 | fat: 5g | protein: 29g | carbs: 25g | sugars: 6g | fiber: 6g | sodium: 495mg

# Easy Southern Brunswick Stew

**Prep time: 20 minutes | Cook time: 8 minutes | Serves 12**

2 pounds (907 g) pork butt, visible fat removed
1 (17-ounce / 482-g) can white corn
1¼ cups ketchup
2 cups diced, cooked potatoes
1 (10-ounce / 283-g) package frozen peas
2 (10¾-ounce / 305-g) cans reduced-sodium tomato soup
Hot sauce to taste, optional

1. Place pork in the Instant Pot and secure the lid.
2. Press the Slow Cook setting and cook on low 6 to 8 hours.
3. When cook time is over, remove the meat from the bone and shred, removing and discarding all visible fat.
4. Combine all the meat and remaining ingredients (except the hot sauce) in the inner pot of the Instant Pot.
5. Secure the lid once more and cook in Slow Cook mode on low for 30 minutes more. Add hot sauce if you wish.

**Per Serving**
calories: 213 | fat: 7g | protein: 13g | carbs: 27g | sugars: 9g | fiber: 3g | sodium: 584mg

# Three-Bean Chili

**Prep time: 30 minutes | Cook time: 15 minutes | Serves 6**

1 pound (454 g) extra-lean ground beef
1 medium onion, diced
1 cup medium salsa
1 package low-sodium dry chili seasoning
1 (16-ounce / 454-g) can low-sodium red kidney beans, drained
1 (16-ounce / 454-g) can low-sodium black beans, drained
1 (16-ounce / 454-g) can low-sodium white kidney, or garbanzo, beans drained
1 (14-ounce / 397-g) can low-sodium crushed tomatoes
1 (14-ounce / 397-g) can low-sodium diced tomatoes
5 drops liquid stevia

1. Turn the Instant Pot to Sauté and add a touch of olive oil or cooking spray to the inner pot. Brown the beef and onion. Press Cancel when done.
2. Stir in the remaining ingredients.
3. Secure the lid and make sure vent is set to sealing. Press Manual and set for 15 minutes.
4. When cooking time is done, let the pressure release naturally for 10 minutes and then manually release the rest.

**Per Serving**
calories: 245 | fat: 8g | protein: 21g | carbs: 22g | sugars: 6g | fiber: 6g | sodium: 589mg

# Pork Chili



1 pound (454 g) boneless pork ribs
2 (14½-ounce / 411-g) cans fire-roasted diced tomatoes
2 (4¼-ounce / 120-g) cans diced green chiles, drained
½ cup chopped onion                                    1 clove garlic, minced
1 tablespoon chili powder

1.  Layer the ingredients into the Instant Pot inner pot in the order given.
2.  Secure the lid. Cook on the high Slow Cook function for 4 hours or on low 6 to 8 hours, or until pork is tender but not dry.
3.  Cut up or shred meat. Stir into the chili and serve.

**Per Serving**
calories: 180 | fat: 7g | protein: 18g | carbs: 12g | sugars: 6g | fiber: 3g | sodium: 495mg

# Vegetarian Chili

**Prep time: 25 minutes | Cook time: 10 minutes | Serves 6**

2 teaspoons olive oil                                  3 garlic cloves, minced
2 onions, chopped                                      1 green bell pepper, chopped
1 cup textured vegetable protein (T.V.P.)
1 (1-pound / 454-g) can beans of your choice, drained
1 jalapeño pepper, seeds removed, chopped
1 (28-ounce / 794-g) can diced Italian tomatoes
1 bay leaf                                             1 tablespoon dried oregano
½ teaspoon salt                                        ¼ teaspoons pepper

1.  Set the Instant Pot to the Sauté function. As it's heating, add the olive oil, garlic, onions, and bell pepper. Stir constantly for about 5 minutes as it all cooks. Press Cancel.
2.  Place all of the remaining ingredients into the inner pot of the Instant pot and stir.
3.  Secure the lid and make sure vent is set to sealing. Cook on Manual mode for 10 minutes.
4.  When cook time is up, let the steam release naturally for 5 minutes and then manually release the rest.

**Per Serving**
calories: 242 | fat: 2g | protein: 17g | carbs: 36g | sugars: 9g | fiber: 12g | sodium: 489mg

# Turkey and Pinto Chili

**Prep time: 10 minutes | Cook time: 1 hour | Serves 8**

2 tablespoons cold-pressed avocado oil

1 large yellow onion, diced

2 carrots, diced

2 teaspoons fine sea salt

2 pounds (907 g) 93 percent lean ground turkey

2 (4-ounce / 113-g) cans fire-roasted diced green chiles

4 tablespoons chili powder

2 teaspoons ground coriander

1 teaspoon dried sage

4 garlic cloves, diced

4 jalapeño chiles, seeded and diced

4 celery stalks, diced

2 teaspoons ground cumin

1 teaspoon dried oregano

1 cup low-sodium chicken broth

3 cups drained cooked pinto beans, or 2 (15-ounce / 425-g) cans pinto beans, drained and rinsed

2 (14½-ounce / 411-g) cans no-salt petite diced tomatoes and their liquid

¼ cup tomato paste

1. Select the Sauté setting on the Instant Pot and heat the oil and garlic for 3 minutes, until the garlic is bubbling but not browned. Add the onion, jalapeños, carrots, celery, and salt and sauté for 5 minutes, until the onion begins to soften. Add the turkey and sauté, using a wooden spoon or spatula to break up the meat as it cooks, for 6 minutes, until cooked through and no streaks of pink remain. Stir in the green chiles, chili powder, cumin, coriander, oregano, sage, and broth, using a wooden spoon or spatula to nudge any browned bits from the bottom of the pot.
2. Pour in the beans in a layer on top of the turkey. Pour in the tomatoes and their liquid and add the tomato paste in a dollop on top. Do not stir in the beans, tomatoes, or tomato paste.
3. Secure the lid and set the Pressure Release to Sealing. Press the Cancel button to reset the cooking program, then select the Manual setting and set the cooking time for 15 minutes at high pressure. (The pot will take about 15 minutes to come up to pressure before the cooking program begins.)
4. When the cooking program ends, let the pressure release naturally for at least 20 minutes, then move the Pressure Release to Venting to release any remaining steam. Open the pot and stir the chili to mix all of the ingredients.
5. Press the Cancel button to reset the cooking program, then select the Sauté setting and set the cooking time for 10 minutes. Allow the chili to reduce and thicken. Do not stir the chili while it is cooking, as this will cause it to sputter more.
6. When the cooking program ends, the pot will turn off. Wearing heat-resistant mitts, remove the inner pot from the housing. Wait for about 2 minutes to allow the chili to stop simmering, then give it a final stir.
7. Ladle the chili into bowls and serve hot.

**Per Serving**

calories: 354 | fat: 14g | protein: 30g | carbs: 28g | sugars: 6g | fiber: 9g | sodium: 819mg

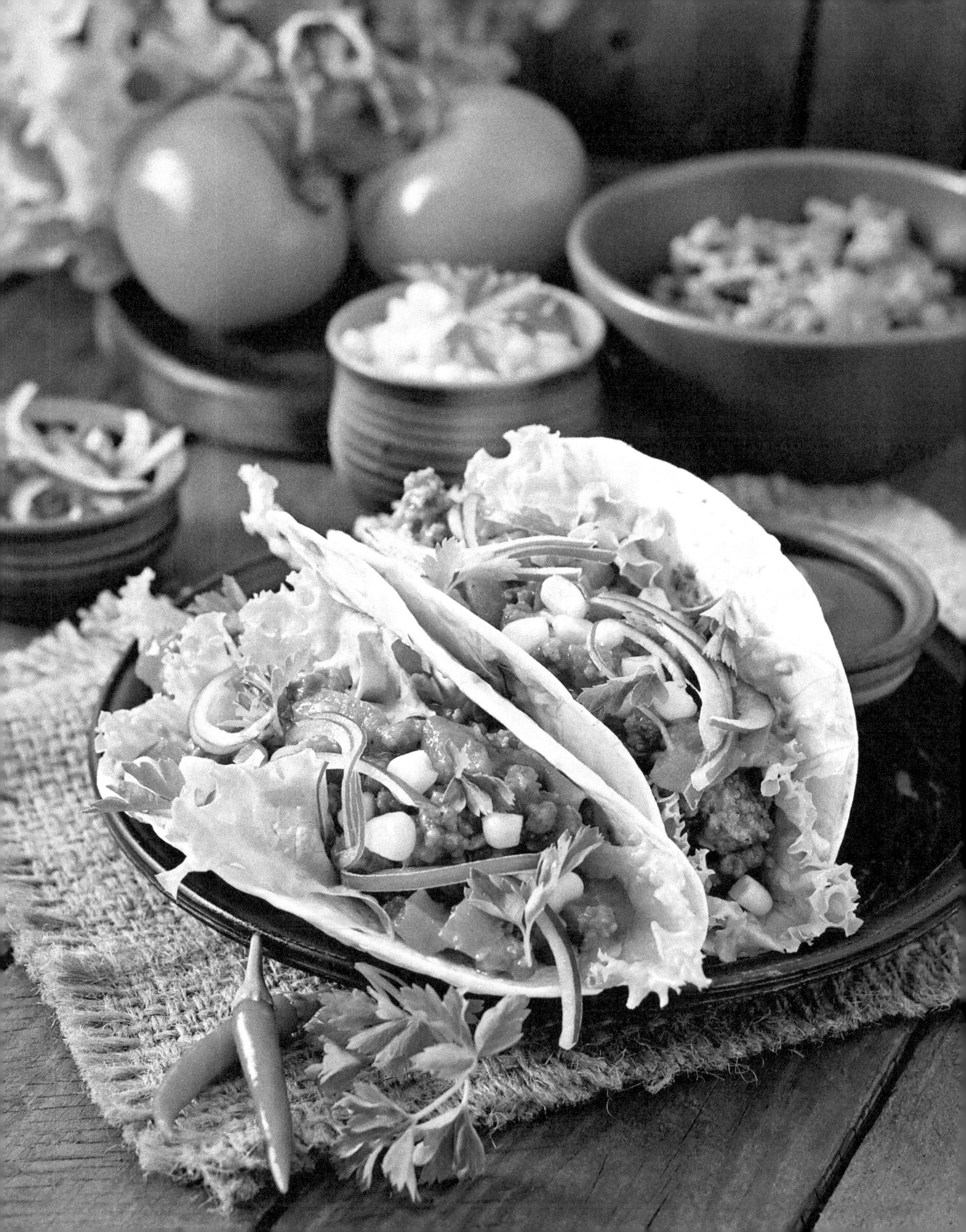

# Chapter 6 Vegetables and Sides

63   Vegetable Medley    56

64   Best Brown Rice    56

65   Vegetable Curry    56

66   Parmesan Cauliflower Mash    57

67   Spaghetti Squash    57

68   Corn on the Cob    58

69   Lemony Brussels Sprouts with Poppy Seeds    58

70   Parmesan-Topped Acorn Squash    59

71   Italian Wild Mushrooms    59

72   Wild Rice Salad with Cranberries and Almonds    60

73   Caramelized Onions    60

74   Potatoes with Parsley    61

75   Perfect Sweet Potatoes    61

# Vegetable Medley

**Prep time: 20 minutes | Cook time: 2 minutes | Serves 8**

2 medium parsnips

1 turnip, about 4½ inches diameter

1 teaspoon salt

2 tablespoons canola or olive oil

4 medium carrots

1 cup water

3 tablespoons sugar

½ teaspoon salt

1. Clean and peel vegetables. Cut in 1-inch pieces.
2. Place the cup of water and 1 teaspoon salt into the Instant Pot's inner pot with the vegetables.
3. Secure the lid and make sure vent is set to sealing. Press Manual and set for 2 minutes.
4. When cook time is up, release the pressure manually and press Cancel. Drain the water from the inner pot.
5. Press Sauté and stir in sugar, oil, and salt. Cook until sugar is dissolved. Serve.

**Per Serving**

calories: 63 | fat: 2g | protein: 1g | carbs: 12g | sugars: 6g | fiber: 2g | sodium: 327mg

# Best Brown Rice

**Prep time: 5 minutes | Cook time: 22 minutes | Serves 6 to 12**

2 cups brown rice

2½ cups water

1. Rinse brown rice in a fine-mesh strainer.
2. Add rice and water to the inner pot of the Instant Pot.
3. Secure the lid and make sure vent is on sealing.
4. Use Manual setting and select 22 minutes and cook on high pressure.
5. When cooking time is done, let the pressure release naturally for 10 minutes, then press Cancel and manually release any remaining pressure.

**Per Serving**

calories: 114 | fat: 1g | protein: 2g | carbs: 23g | sugars: 0g | fiber: 1g | sodium: 3mg

# Vegetable Curry

**Prep time: 25 minutes | Cook time: 3 minutes | Serves 10**

1 (16-ounce / 454-g) package baby carrots

1 pound (454 g) fresh or frozen green beans, cut in 2-inch pieces

1 medium green pepper, chopped

1 to 2 cloves garlic, minced

1 (28-ounce / 794-g) can crushed tomatoes

1½ teaspoons chicken bouillon granules

3 tablespoons minute tapioca

3 medium potatoes, unpeeled, cubed

1 medium onion, chopped

1 (15-ounce / 425-g) can garbanzo beans, drained

3 teaspoons curry powder

1¾ cups boiling water

1. Combine carrots, potatoes, green beans, pepper, onion, garlic, garbanzo beans, crushed tomatoes, and curry powder in the Instant Pot.
2. Dissolve bouillon in boiling water, then stir in tapicoa. Pour over the contents of the Instant Pot and stir.
3. Secure the lid and make sure vent is set to sealing. Press Manual and set for 3 minutes.

4.   When cook time is up, manually release the pressure.

**Per Serving**
calories: 166 | fat: 1g | protein: 6g | carbs: 35g | sugars: 10g | fiber: 8g | sodium: 436mg

# Parmesan Cauliflower Mash

**Prep time: 7 minutes | Cook time: 5 minutes | Serves 4**

1 head cauliflower, cored and cut into large florets
½ teaspoon kosher salt
2 tablespoons plain Greek yogurt
1 tablespoon unsalted butter or ghee (optional)

½ teaspoon garlic pepper
¾ cup freshly grated Parmesan cheese
Chopped fresh chives

1.   Pour 1 cup of water into the electric pressure cooker and insert a steamer basket or wire rack.
2.   Place the cauliflower in the basket.
3.   Close and lock the lid of the pressure cooker. Set the valve to sealing.
4.   Cook on high pressure for 5 minutes.
5.   When the cooking is complete, hit Cancel and quick release the pressure.
6.   Once the pin drops, unlock and remove the lid.
7.   Remove the cauliflower from the pot and pour out the water. Return the cauliflower to the pot and add the salt, garlic pepper, yogurt, and cheese. Use an immersion blender or potato masher to purée or mash the cauliflower in the pot.
8.   Spoon into a serving bowl, and garnish with butter (if using) and chives.

**Per Serving**
calories: 141 | fat: 6g | protein: 12g | carbs: 12g | sugars: 9g | fiber: 4g | sodium: 592mg

# Spaghetti Squash

**Prep time: 5 minutes | Cook time: 7 minutes | Serves 4**

1 spaghetti squash (about 2 pounds / 907 g)

1.   Cut the spaghetti squash in half crosswise and use a large spoon to remove the seeds.
2.   Pour 1 cup of water into the electric pressure cooker and insert a wire rack or trivet.
3.   Place the squash halves on the rack, cut-side up.
4.   Close and lock the lid of the pressure cooker. Set the valve to sealing.
5.   Cook on high pressure for 7 minutes.
6.   When the cooking is complete, hit Cancel and quick release the pressure.
7.   Once the pin drops, unlock and remove the lid.
8.   With tongs, remove the squash from the pot and transfer it to a plate. When it is cool enough to handle, scrape the squash with the tines of a fork to remove the strands. Discard the skin.

**Per Serving**
calories: 10 | fat: 0g | protein: 0g | carbs: 3g | sugars: 1g | fiber: 1g | sodium: 17mg

# Corn on the Cob

**Prep time: 10 minutes | Cook time: 5 minutes | Serves 12**

**6 ears corn**

1. Remove the husks and silk from the corn. Cut or break each ear in half.
2. Pour 1 cup of water into the bottom of the electric pressure cooker. Insert a wire rack or trivet.
3. Place the corn upright on the rack, cut-side down. Close and lock the lid of the pressure cooker. Set the valve to sealing.
4. Cook on high pressure for 5 minutes.
5. When the cooking is complete, hit Cancel and quick release the pressure.
6. Once the pin drops, unlock and remove the lid.
7. Use tongs to remove the corn from the pot. Season as desired and serve immediately.

**Per Serving (½ ear of corn)**
calories: 62 | fat: 1g | protein: 2g | carbs: 14g | sugars: 5g | fiber: 1g | sodium: 11mg

# Lemony Brussels Sprouts with Poppy Seeds

**Prep time: 10 minutes | Cook time: 2 minutes | Serves 4**

**1 pound (454 g) Brussels sprouts**
**2 tablespoons avocado oil, divided**
**1 cup vegetable broth or chicken bone broth**
**1 tablespoon minced garlic**
**Freshly ground black pepper, to taste**
**½ tablespoon poppy seeds**

**½ teaspoon kosher salt**
**½ medium lemon**

1. Trim the Brussels sprouts by cutting off the stem ends and removing any loose outer leaves. Cut each in half lengthwise (through the stem).
2. Set the electric pressure cooker to the Sauté/More setting. When the pot is hot, pour in 1 tablespoon of the avocado oil.
3. Add half of the Brussels sprouts to the pot, cut-side down, and let them brown for 3 to 5 minutes without disturbing. Transfer to a bowl and add the remaining tablespoon of avocado oil and the remaining Brussels sprouts to the pot. Hit Cancel and return all of the Brussels sprouts to the pot.
4. Add the broth, garlic, salt, and a few grinds of pepper. Stir to distribute the seasonings.
5. Close and lock the lid of the pressure cooker. Set the valve to sealing.
6. Cook on high pressure for 2 minutes.
7. While the Brussels sprouts are cooking, zest the lemon, then cut it into quarters.
8. When the cooking is complete, hit Cancel and quick release the pressure.
9. Once the pin drops, unlock and remove the lid.
10. Using a slotted spoon, transfer the Brussels sprouts to a serving bowl. Toss with the lemon zest, a squeeze of lemon juice, and the poppy seeds. Serve immediately.

**Per Serving**
calories: 125 | fat: 8g | protein: 4g | carbs: 13g | sugars: 3g | fiber: 5g | sodium: 504mg

# Parmesan-Topped Acorn Squash

**Prep time: 10 minutes | Cook time: 20 minutes | Serves 4**

1 acorn squash (about 1 pound / 454 g)
1 teaspoon dried sage leaves, crumbled
⅛ teaspoon kosher salt
2 tablespoons freshly grated Parmesan cheese

1 tablespoon extra-virgin olive oil
¼ teaspoon freshly grated nutmeg
⅛ teaspoon freshly ground black pepper

1. Cut the acorn squash in half lengthwise and remove the seeds. Cut each half in half for a total of 4 wedges. Snap off the stem if it's easy to do.
2. In a small bowl, combine the olive oil, sage, nutmeg, salt, and pepper. Brush the cut sides of the squash with the olive oil mixture.
3. Pour 1 cup of water into the electric pressure cooker and insert a wire rack or trivet.
4. Place the squash on the trivet in a single layer, skin-side down.
5. Close and lock the lid of the pressure cooker. Set the valve to sealing.
6. Cook on high pressure for 20 minutes.
7. When the cooking is complete, hit Cancel and quick release the pressure.
8. Once the pin drops, unlock and remove the lid.
9. Carefully remove the squash from the pot, sprinkle with the Parmesan, and serve.

**Per Serving**
calories: 85 | fat: 4g | protein: 2g | carbs: 12g | sugars: 0g | fiber: 2g | sodium: 282mg

# Italian Wild Mushrooms

**Prep time: 30 minutes | Cook time: 3 minutes | Serves 10**

2 tablespoons canola oil
4 garlic cloves, minced
3 large green bell peppers, chopped
1 (12-ounce / 340-g) package oyster mushrooms, cleaned and chopped
3 fresh bay leaves
10 fresh basil leaves, chopped
1 teaspoon salt
1½ teaspoons pepper
1 (28-ounce / 794-g) can Italian plum tomatoes, crushed or chopped

2 large onions, chopped
3 large red bell peppers, chopped

1. Press Sauté on the Instant Pot and add in the oil. Once the oil is heated, add the onions, garlic, peppers, and mushroom to the oil. Sauté just until mushrooms begin to turn brown.
2. Add remaining ingredients. Stir well.
3. Secure the lid and make sure vent is set to sealing. Press Manual and set time for 3 minutes.
4. When cook time is up, release the pressure manually. Discard bay leaves.

**Per Serving**
calories: 82 | fat: 3g | protein: 3g | carbs: 13g | sugars: 8g | fiber: 4g | sodium: 356mg

# Wild Rice Salad with Cranberries and Almonds

**Prep time: 10 minutes | Cook time: 25 minutes | Serves 18**

**Rice:**
2 cups wild rice blend, rinsed
2½ cups vegetable broth or chicken bone broth
1 teaspoon kosher salt
**Dressing:**
¼ cup extra-virgin olive oil
1½ teaspoons grated orange zest
1 teaspoon honey or pure maple syrup
¼ cup white wine vinegar
Juice of 1 medium orange (about ¼ cup)
**Salad:**
¾ cup unsweetened dried cranberries
Freshly ground black pepper, to taste
½ cup sliced almonds, toasted

**Make the Rice**
1. In the electric pressure cooker, combine the rice, salt, and broth.
2. Close and lock the lid. Set the valve to sealing.
3. Cook on high pressure for 25 minutes.
4. When the cooking is complete, hit Cancel and allow the pressure to release naturally for 15 minutes, then quick release any remaining pressure.
5. Once the pin drops, unlock and remove the lid.
6. Let the rice cool briefly, then fluff it with a fork.

**Make the Dressing**
7. While the rice cooks, make the dressing: In a small jar with a screw-top lid, combine the olive oil, vinegar, zest, juice, and honey. (If you don't have a jar, whisk the ingredients together in a small bowl.) Shake to combine.

**Make the Salad**
8. In a large bowl, combine the rice, cranberries, and almonds.
9. Add the dressing and seaso7.

**Per Serving (⅓ cup)**
calories: 126 | fat: 5g | protein: 3g | carbs: 18g | sugars: 2g | fiber: 2g | sodium: 120mg

# Caramelized Onions

**Prep time: 10 minutes | Cook time: 35 minutes | Serves 8**

4 tablespoons margarine
6 large Vidalia or other sweet onions, sliced into thin half rings
1 (10-ounce / 283-g) can chicken or vegetable broth

1. Press Sauté on the Instant Pot. Add in the margarine and let melt.
2. Once the margarine is melted, stir in the onions and sauté for about 5 minutes. Pour in the broth and then press Cancel.
3. Secure the lid and make sure vent is set to sealing. Press Manual and set time for 20 minutes.
4. When cook time is up, release the pressure manually. Remove the lid and press Sauté. Stir the onion mixture for about 10 more minutes, allowing extra liquid to cook off.

**Per Serving**
calories: 123 | fat: 6g | protein: 2g | carbs: 15g | sugars: 10g | fiber: 3g | sodium: 325mg

# Potatoes with Parsley

**Prep time: 10 minutes | Cook time: 5 minutes | Serves 4**

3 tablespoons margarine, divided
2 pounds (907 g) medium red potatoes (about 2 ounces / 57 g each), halved lengthwise
1 clove garlic, minced
½ cup low-sodium chicken broth
½ teaspoon salt
2 tablespoons chopped fresh parsley

1. Place 1 tablespoon margarine in the inner pot of the Instant Pot and select Sauté.
2. After margarine is melted, add potatoes, garlic, and salt, stirring well.
3. Sauté 4 minutes, stirring frequently.
4. Add chicken broth and stir well.
5. Seal lid, make sure vent is on sealing, then select Manual for 5 minutes on high pressure.
6. When cooking time is up, manually release the pressure.
7. Strain potatoes, toss with remaining 2 tablespoons margarine and chopped parsley, and serve immediately.

**Per Serving**
calories: 237 | fat: 9g | protein: 5g | carbs: 37g | sugars: 3g | fiber: 4g | sodium: 389mg

# Perfect Sweet Potatoes

**Prep time: 5 minutes | Cook time: 15 minutes | Serves 4 to 6**

4 to 6 medium sweet potatoes
1 cup water

1. Scrub skin of sweet potatoes with a brush until clean. Pour water into inner pot of the Instant Pot. Place steamer basket in the bottom of the inner pot. Place sweet potatoes on top of steamer basket.
2. Secure the lid and turn valve to seal.
3. Select the Manual mode and set to pressure cook on high for 15 minutes.
4. Allow pressure to release naturally (about 10 minutes).
5. Once the pressure valve lowers, remove lid and serve immediately.

**Per Serving**
calories: 112 | fat: 0g | protein: 2g | carbs: 26g | sugars: 5g | fiber: 4g | sodium: 72mg

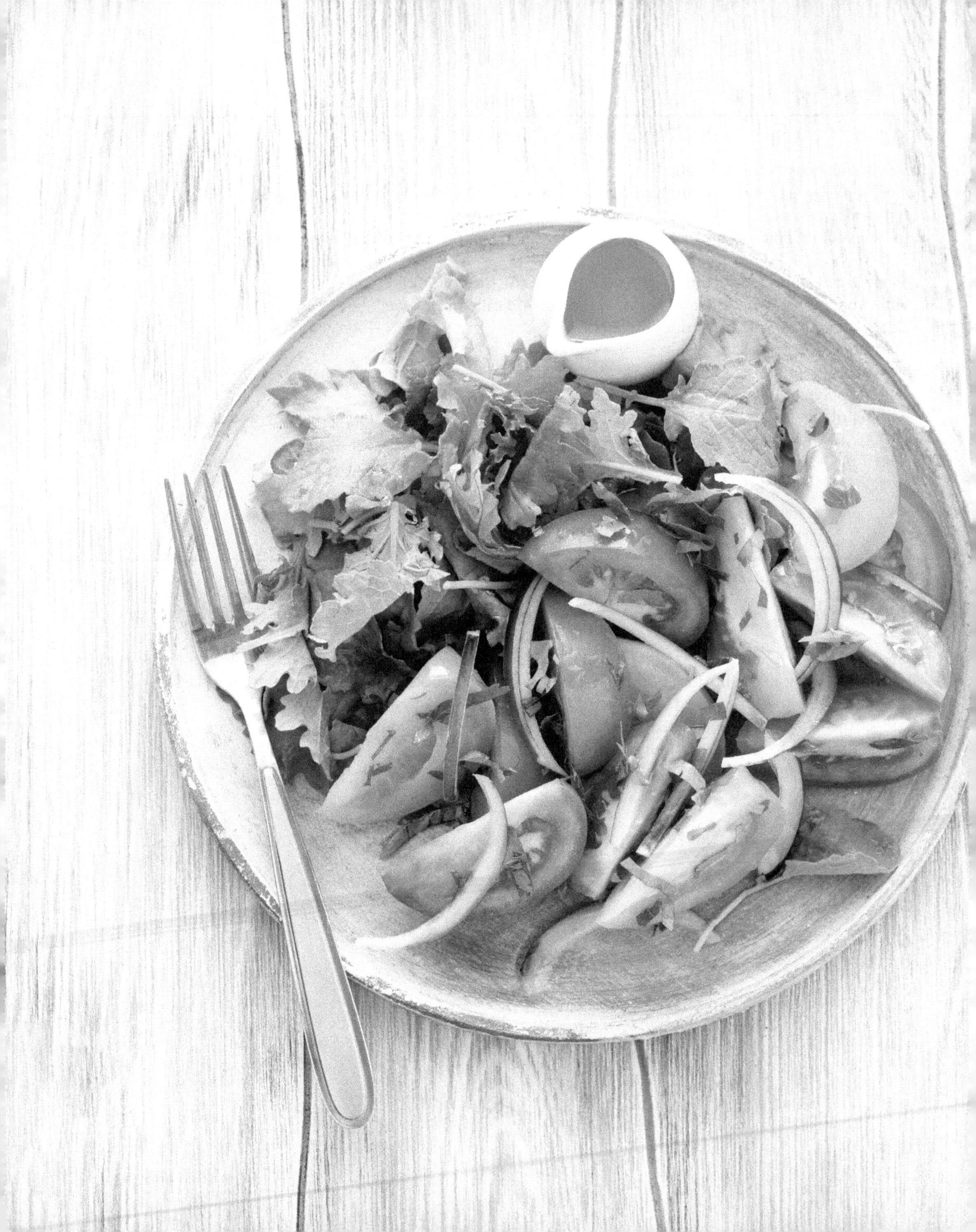

76    Moroccan Eggplant Stew    64

77    Curried Black-Eyed Peas    64

78    Mexican Zucchini Casserole    65

79    Lentils with Carrots    65

80    Butternut Squash Stew with White Beans    66

81    Strawberry Farro Salad    66

82    Palak Tofu    67

83    Chile Relleno Casserole with Salsa Salad    68

84    Pra Ram Vegetables and Peanut Sauce with Seared Tofu    69

85    Lemony Black Rice Salad with Edamame    70

86    15-Bean Pistou Soup    70

87    Minestrone with Red Beans, Zucchini, and Spinach    71

88    Salt-Free No-Soak Beans    72

89    Lentil Sloppy Joes    72

90    Savory Bread Pudding with Mushrooms and Kale    73

91    No-Bake Spaghetti Squash Casserole    74

92    Instant Pot Hoppin' John with Skillet Cauli "Rice"    75

93    Salt-Free Chickpeas (Garbanzo Beans)    76

# Moroccan Eggplant Stew



2 tablespoons avocado oil

2 garlic cloves, minced

¼ teaspoon cayenne pepper

1 cup vegetable broth or water

2 cups chopped eggplant

4 ounces (113 g) tomatillos, husks removed, chopped

1 (14-ounce / 397-g) can diced tomatoes

1 large onion, minced

1 teaspoon ras el hanout spice blend or curry powder

1 teaspoon kosher salt

1 tablespoon tomato paste

2 medium gold potatoes, peeled and chopped

1. Set the electric pressure cooker to the Sauté setting. When the pot is hot, pour in the avocado oil.
2. Sauté the onion for 3 to 5 minutes, until it begins to soften. Add the garlic, ras el hanout, cayenne, and salt. Cook and stir for about 30 seconds. Hit Cancel.
3. Stir in the broth and tomato paste. Add the eggplant, potatoes, tomatillos, and tomatoes with their juices.
4. Close and lock the lid of the pressure cooker. Set the valve to sealing.
5. Cook on high pressure for 3 minutes.
6. When the cooking is complete, hit Cancel and allow the pressure to release naturally.
7. Once the pin drops, unlock and remove the lid.
8. Stir well and spoon into serving bowls.

**Per Serving (1½ cups)**
calories: 216 | fat: 8g | protein: 4g | carbs: 28g | sugars: 8g | fiber: 8g | sodium: 735mg

# Curried Black-Eyed Peas



1 pound (454 g) dried black-eyed peas, rinsed and drained

4 cups vegetable broth

1 cup chopped onion

1½ tablespoons curry powder

1 teaspoon peeled and minced fresh ginger

1 tablespoon extra-virgin olive oil

Lime wedges, for serving

1 cup coconut water

4 large carrots, coarsely chopped

1 tablespoon minced garlic

Kosher salt (optional)

1. In the electric pressure cooker, combine the black-eyed peas, broth, coconut water, onion, carrots, curry powder, garlic, and ginger. Drizzle the olive oil over the top.
2. Close and lock the lid of the pressure cooker. Set the valve to sealing.
3. Cook on high pressure for 25 minutes.
4. When the cooking is complete, hit Cancel and allow the pressure to release naturally for 10 minutes, then quick release any remaining pressure.
5. Once the pin drops, unlock and remove the lid.
6. Season with salt (if using) and squeeze some fresh lime juice on each serving.

**Per Serving (½ cup)**
calories: 112 | fat: 3g | protein: 10g | carbs: 31g | sugars: 6g | fiber: 6g | sodium: 670mg

# Mexican Zucchini Casserole

**Prep time: 15 minutes | Cook time: 15 minutes | Serves 4**

1 (6- to 7-inch) zucchini, trimmed

Nonstick cooking spray

1 (15-ounce / 425-g) can pinto beans, rinsed and drained

1⅓ cups salsa

1⅓ cups shredded Mexican cheese blend

1. Slice the zucchini into rounds. You'll need at least 16 slices.
2. Spray a 6-inch cake pan with nonstick spray.
3. Put the beans into a medium bowl and mash some of them with a fork.
4. Cover the bottom of the pan with about 4 zucchini slices. Add about ⅓ of the beans, ⅓ cup of salsa, and ⅓ cup of cheese. Press down. Repeat for 2 more layers. Add the remaining zucchini, salsa, and cheese. (There are no beans in the top layer.)
5. Cover the pan loosely with foil.
6. Pour 1 cup of water into the electric pressure cooker.
7. Place the pan on the wire rack and carefully lower it into the pot. Close and lock the lid of the pressure cooker. Set the valve to sealing.
8. Cook on high pressure for 15 minutes.
9. When the cooking is complete, hit Cancel and allow the pressure to release naturally.
10. Once the pin drops, unlock and remove the lid.
11. Carefully remove the pan from the pot, lifting by the handles of the wire rack. Let the casserole sit for 5 minutes before slicing into quarters and serving.

**Per Serving**

calories: 252 | fat: 12g | protein: 16g | carbs: 23g | sugars: 4g | fiber: 7g | sodium: 1089mg

# Lentils with Carrots

**Prep time: 15 minutes | Cook time: 12 minutes | Serves 6**

2 tablespoons avocado oil

1 medium onion, chopped

3 celery stalks, chopped

1 teaspoon herbes de Provence

2 large carrots, chopped

2 cups vegetable broth or water

1 cup dried brown or green lentils, rinsed and drained

Kosher salt, to taste

Freshly ground black pepper, to taste

1. Set the electric pressure cooker to the Sauté setting. When the pot is hot, pour in the avocado oil.
2. Sauté the onion and celery for 3 to 5 minutes, until the vegetables begin to soften. Stir in the herbes de Provence and carrots. Hit Cancel. Stir in the broth and lentils.
3. Close and lock the lid of the pressure cooker. Set the valve to sealing.
4. Cook on high pressure for 12 minutes.
5. When the cooking is complete, hit Cancel and allow the pressure to release naturally for 10 minutes, then quick release any remaining pressure.
6. Once the pin drops, unlock and remove the lid.
7. Season with salt and pepper, spoon into bowls, and serve.

**Per Serving (⅔ cup)**

calories: 178 | fat: 5g | protein: 9g | carbs: 24g | sugars: 3g | fiber: 11g | sodium: 45mg

# Butternut Squash Stew with White Beans

**Prep time: 16 minutes | Cook time: 7 minutes | Serves 6**

1 pound (454 g) butternut squash, peeled, seeded, and cut into 1-inch cubes (about 3 cups)
1 tablespoon extra-virgin olive oil
1 tablespoon chili powder
1 teaspoon dried oregano
1 teaspoon ground cumin
1 tablespoon garlic pepper or garlic powder
½ teaspoon kosher salt
2 tablespoons finely chopped poblano chile or green bell pepper
3 cups vegetable broth or water
1 (15-ounce / 425-g) can diced tomatoes
1 (15-ounce / 425-g) can white beans, rinsed and drained
1 avocado, chopped just before serving

1.  In the electric pressure cooker, toss the squash with the olive oil, chili powder, oregano, cumin, garlic pepper, and salt.
2.  Stir in the poblano, broth, and tomatoes and their juices.
3.  Close and lock the lid of the pressure cooker. Set the valve to sealing.
4.  Cook on high pressure for 7 minutes.
5.  When the cooking is complete, hit Cancel and quick release the pressure.
6.  Once the pin drops, unlock and remove the lid.
7.  Stir in the beans and let the stew sit for about 5 minutes to let the beans warm up.
8.  Use an immersion blender to purée about one-third of the stew right in the pot. (I like to leave some chunks of squash and whole beans for more texture.)
9.  Spoon into serving bowls and top with the avocado.

**Per Serving (1 cup)**
calories: 196 | fat: 6g | protein: 7g | carbs: 31g | sugars: 4g | fiber: 8g | sodium: 332mg

# Strawberry Farro Salad

**Prep time: 17 minutes | Cook time: 10 minutes | Serves 8**

**Farro:**
1 cup farro, rinsed and drained
¼ teaspoon kosher salt
**Dressing:**
1 tablespoon freshly squeezed lime juice (from ½ medium lime)
½ tablespoon fruit-flavored balsamic vinegar
½ teaspoon Dijon mustard
½ tablespoon honey or pure maple syrup
½ teaspoon poppy seeds
¼ cup extra-virgin olive oil
**Salad:**
1¼ cups sliced strawberries
¼ cup slivered almonds, toasted
Freshly ground black pepper, to taste
Fresh basil leaves, cut into a chiffonade, for garnish

**Make the Farro**
1.  In the electric pressure cooker, combine the farro, salt, and 2 cups of water.
2.  Close and lock the lid. Set the valve to sealing.
3.  Cook on high pressure for 10 minutes.
4.  When the cooking is complete, allow the pressure to release naturally for 10 minutes, then quick release the remaining pressure. Hit Cancel.

5.    Once the pin drops, unlock and remove the lid.
6.    Fluff the farro with a fork and let cool.

**Make the Dressing**

7.    While the farro is cooking, in a small jar with a screw-top lid, combine the lime juice, balsamic vinegar, mustard, honey, poppy seeds, and olive oil. Shake until well combined.

**Make the Salad**

8.    In a large bowl, toss the farro with the dressing. Stir in the strawberries and almonds.
9.    Season with pepper, garnish with basil, and serve.

**Per Serving (½ cup)**
calories: 176 | fat: 9g | protein: 3g | carbs: 22g | sugars: 3g | fiber: 2g | sodium: 68mg

# Palak Tofu

**Prep time: 5 minutes | Cook time: 40 minutes | Serves 4**

1 (14-ounce / 397-g) package extra-firm tofu, drained
5 tablespoons cold-pressed avocado oil
1 yellow onion, diced
3 garlic cloves, minced
½ teaspoon freshly ground black pepper
1 (16-ounce / 454-g) bag frozen chopped spinach
1 (14½-ounce / 411-g) can fire-roasted diced tomatoes and their liquid
¼ cup coconut milk
Cooked brown rice or cauliflower "rice" or whole-grain flatbread, for serving

1-inch piece fresh ginger, peeled and minced
1 teaspoon fine sea salt
¼ teaspoon cayenne pepper
⅓ cup water
2 teaspoons garam masala

1.    Cut the tofu crosswise into eight ½-inch-thick slices. Sandwich the slices between double layers of paper towels or a folded kitchen towel and press firmly to wick away as much moisture as possible. Cut the slices into ½-inch cubes.
2.    Select the Sauté setting on the Instant Pot and and heat 4 tablespoons of the oil for 2 minutes. Add the onion and sauté for about 10 minutes, until it begins to brown.
3.    While the onion is cooking in the Instant Pot, in a large nonstick skillet over medium-high heat, warm the remaining 1 tablespoon oil. Add the tofu in a single layer and cook without stirring for about 3 minutes, until lightly browned.
4.    Using a spatula, turn the cubes over and cook for about 3 minutes more, until browned on the other side. Remove from the heat and set aside.
5.    Add the ginger and garlic to the onion in the Instant Pot and sauté for about 2 minutes, until the garlic is bubbling but not browned. Add the sautéed tofu, salt, black pepper, and cayenne and stir gently to combine, taking care not to break up the tofu. Add the spinach and stir gently. Pour in the water and then pour the tomatoes and their liquid over the top in an even layer. Do not stir them in.
6.    Secure the lid and set the Pressure Release to Sealing. Press the Cancel button to reset the cooking program, then select the Manual setting and set the cooking time for 10 minutes at low pressure. (The pot will take about 15 minutes to come up to pressure before the cooking program begins.)
7.    When the cooking program ends, let the pressure release naturally for 10 minutes, then move the Pressure Release to Venting to release any remaining steam. Open the pot, add the coconut milk and garam masala, and stir to combine.
8.    Ladle the tofu onto plates or into bowls. Serve piping hot, with the "rice" alongside.

**Per Serving**
calories: 345 | fat: 24g | protein: 14g | carbs: 18g | sugars: 5g | fiber: 6g | sodium: 777mg

# Chile Relleno Casserole with Salsa Salad

**Prep time: 10 minutes | Cook time: 55 minutes | Serves 4**

**Casserole:**
½ cup gluten-free flour
1 teaspoon baking powder
6 large eggs
½ cup nondairy milk or whole milk
3 (4-ounce / 113-g) cans fire-roasted diced green chiles, drained
1 cup nondairy cheese shreds or shredded Mozzarella cheese
**Salad:**
1 head green leaf lettuce, shredded
2 Roma tomatoes, seeded and diced
1 green bell pepper, seeded and diced
½ small yellow onion, diced
1 jalapeño chile, seeded and diced (optional)
2 tablespoons chopped fresh cilantro
4 teaspoons extra-virgin olive oil
4 teaspoons fresh lime juice
⅛ teaspoon fine sea salt

1. To make the casserole: Pour 1 cup water into the Instant Pot. Butter a 7-cup round heatproof glass dish or coat with nonstick cooking spray and place the dish on a long-handled silicone steam rack. (If you don't have the long-handled rack, use the wire metal steam rack and a homemade sling)
2. In a medium bowl, whisk together the flour and baking powder. Add the eggs and milk and whisk until well blended, forming a batter. Stir in the chiles and ¾ cup of the cheese.
3. Pour the batter into the prepared dish and cover tightly with aluminum foil. Holding the handles of the steam rack, lower the dish into the Instant Pot.
4. Secure the lid and set the Pressure Release to Sealing. Select the Manual setting and set the cooking time for 40 minutes at high pressure. (The pot will take about 10 minutes to come up to pressure before the cooking program begins.)
5. When the cooking program ends, let the pressure release naturally for at least 10 minutes, then move the Pressure Release to Venting to release any remaining steam. Open the pot and, wearing heat-resistant mitts, grasp the handles of the steam rack and lift it out of the pot. Uncover the dish, taking care not to get burned by the steam or to drip condensation onto the casserole. While the casserole is still piping hot, sprinkle the remaining ¼ cup cheese evenly on top. Let the cheese melt for 5 minutes.
6. To make the salad: While the cheese is melting, in a large bowl, combine the lettuce, tomatoes, bell pepper, onion, jalapeño (if using), cilantro, oil, lime juice, and salt. Toss until evenly combined.
7. Cut the casserole into wedges. Serve warm, with the salad on the side.

**Per Serving**
calories: 361 | fat: 22g | protein: 21g | carbs: 23g | sugars: 8g | fiber: 3g | sodium: 421mg

# Pra Ram Vegetables and Peanut Sauce with Seared Tofu

**Prep time: 5 minutes | Cook time: 20 minutes | Serves 4**

**Peanut Sauce:**

2 tablespoons cold-pressed avocado oil

½ cup creamy natural peanut butter

2 tablespoons brown rice syrup

1 tablespoon plus 1 teaspoon soy sauce, tamari, or coconut aminos

¼ cup water

2 garlic cloves, minced

½ cup coconut milk

**Vegetables:**

2 carrots, sliced on the diagonal ¼ inch thick

8 ounces (227 g) zucchini, julienned ¼ inch thick

1 pound (454 g) broccoli florets

½ small head green cabbage, cut into 1-inch-thick wedges (with core intact so wedges hold together)

**Tofu:**

1 (14-ounce / 397-g) package extra-firm tofu, drained

¼ teaspoon fine sea salt

1 tablespoon cornstarch

¼ teaspoon freshly ground black pepper

2 tablespoons coconut oil

1. To make the peanut sauce: In a small saucepan over medium heat, warm the oil and garlic for about 2 minutes, until the garlic is bubbling but not browned. Add the peanut butter, coconut milk, brown rice syrup, soy sauce, and water; stir to combine; and bring to a simmer (this will take about 3 minutes). As soon as the mixture is fully combined and at a simmer, remove from the heat and keep warm. The peanut sauce will keep in an airtight container in the refrigerator for up to 5 days.

2. To make the vegetables: Pour 1 cup water into the Instant Pot and place a steamer basket into the pot. In order, layer the carrots, zucchini, broccoli, and cabbage in the steamer basket, finishing with the cabbage.

3. Secure the lid and set the Pressure Release to Sealing. Select the Steam setting and set the cooking time for 0 (zero) minutes at low pressure. (The pot will take about 15 minutes to come up to pressure before the cooking program begins.)

4. To prepare the tofu: While the vegetables are steaming, cut the tofu crosswise into eight ½-inch-thick slices. Cut each of the slices in half crosswise, creating squares. Sandwich the squares between double layers of paper towels or a folded kitchen towel and press firmly to wick away as much moisture as possible. Sprinkle the tofu squares on both sides with the salt and pepper, then sprinkle them on both sides with the cornstarch. Using your fingers, spread the cornstarch on the top and bottom of each square to coat evenly.

5. In a large nonstick skillet over medium-high heat, warm the oil for about 3 minutes, until shimmering. Add the tofu and sear, turning once, for about 6 minutes per side, until crispy and golden. Divide the tofu evenly among four plates.

6. When the cooking program ends, perform a quick pressure release by moving the Pressure Release to Venting. Open the pot and, wearing heat-resistant mitts, grasp the handles of the steamer basket and lift it out of the pot.

7. Divide the vegetables among the plates, arranging them around the tofu. Spoon the peanut sauce over the tofu and serve.

**Per Serving**

calories: 380 | fat: 22g | protein: 18g | carbs: 30g | sugars: 9g | fiber: 10g | sodium: 381mg

# Lemony Black Rice Salad with Edamame



**Rice:**
1 cup black rice (forbidden rice), rinsed and still wet
**Dressing:**
3 tablespoons extra-virgin olive oil

2 tablespoons freshly squeezed lemon juice

2 tablespoons white wine vinegar or rice vinegar
1 tablespoon honey or pure maple syrup

1 tablespoon sesame oil

**Salad:**
1 (8-ounce / 227-g) bag frozen shelled edamame, thawed (about 1½ cups)
2 scallions, both white and green parts, thinly sliced
¼ cup chopped walnuts

Kosher salt, to taste

Freshly ground black pepper, to taste

### Make the Rice
1. In the electric pressure cooker, combine the rice and 1 cup of water.
2. Close and lock the lid of the pressure cooker. Set the valve to sealing.
3. Cook on high pressure for 22 minutes.
4. When the cooking is complete, hit Cancel and allow the pressure to release naturally for 10 minutes, then quick release any remaining pressure.
5. Once the pin drops, unlock and remove the lid.
6. Fluff the rice with a fork and let it cool.

### Make the Dressing
7. While the rice is cooking, make the dressing. In a small jar with a screw-top lid, combine the olive oil, lemon juice, vinegar, honey or maple syrup, and sesame oil. Shake until well combined.

### Make the Salad
8. Shake up the dressing. In a large bowl, toss the rice and dressing. Stir in the edamame, scallions, and walnuts.
9. Season with salt and pepper.

**Per Serving (½ cup)**
calories: 170 | fat: 11g | protein: 5g | carbs: 15g | sugars: 3g | fiber: 2g | sodium: 10mg

# 15-Bean Pistou Soup



10 ounces (283 g) 15-Bean Soup mix, beans only, rinsed and drained (half of a 20-ounce / 567-g bag)
4 cups vegetable broth or water

½ cup chopped onion

½ cup chopped green bell pepper

1 celery stalk, chopped

1 tablespoon minced garlic

½ teaspoon Italian seasoning

1 bay leaf

1 tablespoon extra-virgin olive oil

2 tablespoons tomato paste

6 tablespoons store-bought pesto

1. In the electric pressure cooker, combine the beans, broth, onion, bell pepper, celery, garlic, Italian seasoning, and bay leaf. Drizzle the olive oil over the top. (The oil will help control the foam produced by the cooking beans.)
2. Close and lock the lid of the pressure cooker. Set the valve to sealing.

3. Cook on high pressure for 45 minutes.
4. When the cooking is complete, hit Cancel. Allow the pressure to release naturally for 20 minutes, then quick release any remaining pressure.
5. Once the pin drops, unlock and remove the lid.
6. Stir in the tomato paste and hit Sauté. Cook for about 5 minutes or until the soup thickens. Discard the bay leaf.
7. Spoon into serving bowls and top each with 1 tablespoon of pesto.

**Per Serving (1 cup)**
calories: 292 | fat: 13g | protein: 13g | carbs: 34g | sugars: 3g | fiber: 8g | sodium: 125mg

# Minestrone with Red Beans, Zucchini, and Spinach

**Prep time: 15 minutes | Cook time: 5 minutes | Serves 8**

**Soup:**
2 tablespoons avocado oil
1 cup chopped onion
1 celery stalk, chopped
1 teaspoon dried thyme
½ teaspoon dried sage leaves
½ teaspoon freshly ground black pepper
2 cups vegetable broth or water
1 (28-ounce / 794-g) carton or can chopped tomatoes
1 (15-ounce / 425-g) can small red beans, rinsed and drained
2 carrots, peeled and chopped
2 bay leaves
½ cup whole wheat orzo, uncooked (optional)
**Finish:**
1 medium zucchini, quartered lengthwise, then chopped
2 cups baby spinach
¼ cup freshly grated Parmesan cheese
Chopped fresh basil (optional)

**Make the Soup**
1. Set the electric pressure cooker to the Sauté setting. When the pot is hot, pour in the avocado oil.
2. Sauté the onion and celery for 3 to 5 minutes, or until the vegetables begin to soften. Stir in the thyme, sage, and pepper. Hit Cancel.
3. Add the broth, tomatoes and their juices, beans, carrots, bay leaves, and orzo (if using).
4. Close and lock the lid of the pressure cooker. Set the valve to sealing.
5. Cook on high pressure for 5 minutes.
6. When the cooking is complete, hit Cancel and quick release the pressure.
7. Once the pin drops, unlock and remove the lid.
**Finish the Soup**
8. Stir in the zucchini and spinach. Replace the lid and let the pot sit for 10 minutes.
9. Spoon into serving bowls and top with the Parmesan cheese and basil (if using).

**Per Serving (1 cup)**
calories: 152 | fat: 5g | protein: 6g | carbs: 23g | sugars: 8g | fiber: 7g | sodium: 357mg

# Salt-Free No-Soak Beans

**Prep time: 2 minutes | Cook time: 35 minutes | Makes 6 cups**

1 pound (454 g) dried beans, rinsed (unsoaked)
1 tablespoon extra-virgin olive oil

5 cups vegetable broth, chicken bone broth, or water

1. In the electric pressure cooker, combine the beans and broth. Drizzle the oil on top. (The oil will help control the foam produced by the cooking beans.)
2. Close and lock the lid of the pressure cooker. Set the valve to sealing.
3. For black beans, cook on high pressure for 25 minutes.
4. For pinto beans, navy beans, or great northern beans, cook on high pressure for 30 minutes.
5. For cannellini beans, cook on high pressure for 40 minutes.
6. When the cooking is complete, hit Cancel and allow the pressure to release naturally for 20 minutes, then quick release any remaining pressure.
7. Once the pin drops, unlock and remove the lid.
8. Let the beans cool, then pack them into containers and cover with the cooking liquid. Refrigerate for 3 to 5 days or freeze for up to 8 months.

**Per Serving (½ cup)**
calories: 141 | fat: 2g | protein: 8g | carbs: 24g | sugars: 1g | fiber: 6g | sodium: 5mg

# Lentil Sloppy Joes

**Prep time: 15 minutes | Cook time: 40 minutes | Serves 6**

**Sloppy Joes:**
4 tablespoons extra-virgin olive oil
1 yellow onion, diced
1 carrot, diced
1 small Fuji or Gala apple, peeled and grated
1 teaspoon chili powder
½ teaspoon fine sea salt
1 tablespoon Worcestershire sauce
2 cups low-sodium vegetable broth
1 (8-ounce / 227-g) can tomato sauce

2 garlic cloves, minced
1 red bell pepper, diced
2 celery stalks, diced

½ teaspoon smoked paprika
¼ teaspoon freshly ground black pepper
1 tablespoon balsamic vinegar
1⅛ cups green lentils
3 tablespoons tomato paste

**Mushrooms:**
6 portobello mushrooms, stemmed
½ teaspoon fine sea salt

2 tablespoons extra-virgin olive oil
¼ teaspoon freshly ground black pepper

Thin yellow onion slices, for serving

1. To make the Sloppy Joes: Select the Sauté setting on the Instant Pot and heat the oil and garlic for 2 minutes, until the garlic is bubbling but not browned. Add the onion, bell pepper, carrot, and celery and sauté for about 5 minutes, until the onion begins to soften. Add the apple, chili powder, paprika, salt, pepper, Worcestershire sauce, vinegar, broth, and lentils and stir well. Pour in the tomato sauce and dollop the tomato paste on top. Do not stir them in.
2. Secure the lid and set the Pressure Release to Sealing. Press the Cancel button to reset the cooking program, then select the Bean/Chili or Manual setting and set the cooking time for 25 minutes at high pressure. (The

pot will take about 10 minutes to come up to pressure before the cooking program begins.)

3. To cook the mushrooms: While the Sloppy Joes are cooking, position an oven rack 4 to 6 inches below the heat source and preheat the broiler. Line a sheet pan with aluminum foil.
4. Brush both sides of each mushroom with the oil, then sprinkle both sides with the salt and pepper. Place the mushrooms, gill-side down, on the prepared pan. Broil for about 7 minutes, until the mushrooms are a bit softened. Turn off the broiler and leave them in the oven to stay warm and continue cooking a bit from the residual heat.
5. When the cooking program ends, let the pressure release naturally for at least 10 minutes, then move the Pressure Release to Venting to release any remaining steam. Open the pot and stir to combine all of the ingredients.
6. Place the mushrooms, gill-side up, on six plates and ladle the Sloppy Joe mixture over the mushrooms. Top with the onion slices and serve hot.

**Per Serving**
calories: 279 | fat: 14g | protein: 13g | carbs: 37g | sugars: 9g | fiber: 15g | sodium: 660mg

## Savory Bread Pudding with Mushrooms and Kale

**Prep time: 20 minutes | Cook time: 8 minutes | Serves 2**

1 large egg

½ cup 2% milk

½ teaspoon Dijon mustard

Pinch freshly grated nutmeg

Pinch kosher salt

Pinch freshly ground black pepper

1 slice sourdough bread (about 1 ounce / 28 g), cut into 1-inch cubes

1 tablespoon avocado oil

¼ cup chopped onion

2 ounces (57 g) mushrooms, sliced (about 3 creminis)

¼ teaspoon dried thyme

1 cup chopped lacinato kale, stems and ribs removed (from 2 stems)

Nonstick cooking spray

¼ cup grated Gruyère cheese

1 tablespoon shredded Parmesan

1. In a 2-cup measuring cup with a spout, whisk together the egg, milk, mustard, nutmeg, salt, and pepper. Add the bread and submerge it in the liquid.
2. Set the electric pressure cooker to the Sauté setting. When the pot is hot, pour in the avocado oil.
3. Add the onion, mushrooms, and thyme to the pot and sauté for 3 to 5 minutes or until the onion begins to soften. Stir in the kale and cook for about 2 minutes or until it wilts. Hit Cancel.
4. Spray the ramekins with cooking spray. Divide the mushroom mixture between the ramekins. Top each with 2 tablespoons Gruyère. Pour half of the egg mixture into each ramekin and stir. Make sure the bread stays submerged. Cover with foil.
5. Pour 1 cup of water into the electric pressure cooker and insert a wire rack or trivet. Place the ramekins on the rack.
6. Close and lock the lid of the pressure cooker. Set the valve to sealing.
7. Cook on high pressure for 8 minutes.
8. When the cooking is complete, hit Cancel. Allow the pressure to release naturally for 10 minutes, then quick release any remaining pressure.
9. Using tongs or the handles of the rack, transfer the ramekins to a cutting board. Carefully lift the foil and sprinkle the Parmesan on top. Replace the foil for about 5 minutes or until the cheese melts.
10. Remove the foil and serve immediately.

**Per Serving**
calories: 295 | fat: 17g | protein: 13g | carbs: 23g | sugars: 7g | fiber: 3g | sodium: 313mg

# No-Bake Spaghetti Squash Casserole

**Prep time: 10 minutes | Cook time: 45 minutes | Serves 6**

**Marinara:**

3 tablespoons extra-virgin olive oil

1 (28-ounce / 794-g) can whole San Marzano tomatoes and their liquid

2 teaspoons Italian seasoning

½ teaspoon red pepper flakes (optional)

3 garlic cloves, minced

1 teaspoon fine sea salt

**Vegan Parmesan:**

½ cup raw whole cashews

½ teaspoon garlic powder

2 tablespoons nutritional yeast

½ teaspoon fine sea salt

**Vegan Ricotta:**

1 (14-ounce / 397-g) package firm tofu, drained

½ cup raw whole cashews, soaked in water to cover for 1 to 2 hours and then drained

3 tablespoons nutritional yeast

2 tablespoons extra-virgin olive oil

1 teaspoon finely grated lemon zest, plus 2 tablespoons fresh lemon juice

½ cup firmly packed fresh flat-leaf parsley leaves

1 teaspoon garlic powder

½ teaspoon freshly ground black pepper

1½ teaspoons Italian seasoning

1 teaspoon fine sea salt

1 (3½-pound / 1.6-kg) steamed spaghetti squash

2 tablespoons chopped fresh flat-leaf parsley

1. To make the marinara: Select the Sauté setting on the Instant Pot and heat the oil and garlic for about 2 minutes, until the garlic is bubbling but not browned. Add the tomatoes and their liquid and use a wooden spoon or spatula to crush the tomatoes against the side of the pot. Stir in the Italian seasoning, salt, and pepper flakes (if using) and cook, stirring occasionally, for about 10 minutes, until the sauce has thickened a bit. Press the Cancel button to turn off the pot and let the sauce cook from the residual heat for about 5 minutes more, until it is no longer simmering. Wearing heat-resistant mitts, lift the pot out of the housing, pour the sauce into a medium heatproof bowl, and set aside. (You can make the sauce up to 4 days in advance, then let it cool, transfer it to an airtight container, and refrigerate.)
2. To make the vegan Parmesan: In a food processor, combine the cashews, nutritional yeast, garlic powder, and salt. Using 1-second pulses, pulse about ten times, until the mixture resembles grated Parmesan cheese. Transfer to a small bowl and set aside. Do not wash the food processor bowl and blade.
3. To make the vegan ricotta: Cut the tofu crosswise into eight ½-inch-thick slices. Sandwich the slices between double layers of paper towels or a folded kitchen towel and press gently to remove excess moisture. Add the tofu to the food processor along with the cashews, nutritional yeast, oil, lemon zest, lemon juice, parsley, Italian seasoning, garlic powder, salt, and pepper. Process for about 1 minute, until the mixture is mostly smooth with flecks of parsley throughout. Set aside.
4. Return the marinara to the pot. Select the Sauté setting and heat the marinara sauce for about 3 minutes, until it starts to simmer. Add the spaghetti squash and vegan ricotta to the pot and stir to combine. Continue to heat, stirring often, for 8 to 10 minutes, until piping hot. Press the Cancel button to turn off the pot.
5. Spoon the spaghetti squash into bowls, top with the vegan Parmesan and parsley, and serve right away.

**Per Serving**

calories: 307 | fat: 17g | protein: 16g | carbs: 25g | sugars: 2g | fiber: 5g | sodium: 985mg

# Instant Pot Hoppin' John with Skillet Cauli "Rice"

**Prep time: 20 minutes | Cook time: 30 minutes | Serves 6**

**Hoppin' John:**
1 pound (454 g) dried black-eyed peas (about 2¼ cups)
8⅔ cups water
1½ teaspoons fine sea salt
2 tablespoons extra-virgin olive oil
2 garlic cloves, minced
8 ounces (227 g) shiitake mushrooms, stemmed and chopped, or cremini mushrooms, chopped
1 small yellow onion, diced
1 green bell pepper, seeded and diced
2 celery stalks, diced
2 jalapeño chiles, seeded and diced
½ teaspoon smoked paprika
½ teaspoon dried thyme
½ teaspoon dried sage
¼ teaspoon cayenne pepper
2 cups low-sodium vegetable broth
**Cauli "Rice":**
1 tablespoon vegan buttery spread or unsalted butter
1 pound (454 g) riced cauliflower
½ teaspoon fine sea salt

2 green onions, white and green parts, sliced
Hot sauce (such as Tabasco or Crystal), for serving

1.  To make the Hoppin' John: In a large bowl, combine the black-eyed peas, 8 cups of the water, and 1 teaspoon of the salt and stir to dissolve the salt. Let soak for at least 8 hours or up to overnight.
2.  Select the Sauté setting on the Instant Pot and heat the oil and garlic for 3 minutes, until the garlic is bubbling but not browned. Add the mushrooms and the remaining ½ teaspoon salt and sauté for 5 minutes, until the mushrooms have wilted and begun to give up their liquid. Add the onion, bell pepper, celery, and jalapeños and sauté for 4 minutes, until the onion is softened. Add the paprika, thyme, sage, and cayenne and sauté for 1 minute.
3.  Drain the black-eyed peas and add them to the pot along with the broth and remaining ⅔ cup water. The liquid should just barely cover the beans. (Add an additional splash of water if needed.)
4.  Secure the lid and set the Pressure Release to Sealing. Press the Cancel button to reset the cooking program, then select the Bean/Chili or Manual setting and set the cooking time for 5 minutes at high pressure. (The pot will take about 10 minutes to come up to pressure before the cooking program begins.)
5.  When the cooking program ends, let the pressure release naturally for 10 minutes, then move the Pressure Release to Venting to release any remaining steam.
6.  To make the cauli "rice": While the pressure is releasing, in a large skillet over medium heat, melt the buttery spread. Add the cauliflower and salt and sauté for 3 to 5 minutes, until cooked through and piping hot. (If using frozen riced cauliflower, this may take another 2 minutes or so.)
7.  Spoon the cauli "rice" onto individual plates. Open the pot and spoon the black-eyed peas on top of the cauli "rice". Sprinkle with the green onions and serve right away, with the hot sauce on the side.

**Per Serving**
calories: 287 | fat: 7g | protein: 23g | carbs: 56g | sugars: 8g | fiber: 24g | sodium: 894mg

# Salt-Free Chickpeas (Garbanzo Beans)

**Prep time: 5 minutes | Cook time: 35 minutes | Makes 6 cups**

**1 pound (454 g) dried chickpeas**
**2 bay leaves**
**Fresh herbs, like parsley, thyme, rosemary, etc., cut into 3-inch pieces and tied together with kitchen twine (optional)**

1. Rinse the chickpeas and put them in the electric pressure cooker. Add 8 cups of water, the bay leaves, and the herbs (if using).
2. Close and lock the lid. Turn the pressure valve to sealing.
3. Cook on high pressure for 35 minutes.
4. When the cooking is complete, hit Cancel. Allow the pressure to release naturally for 20 minutes, then quick release any remaining pressure.
5. Unlock and remove the lid. Discard the bay leaves and herb bundle.
6. Transfer the chickpeas to storage containers, covered with the cooking liquid, and let cool. Refrigerate for 3 or 4 days or freeze for up to 6 months.

**Per Serving (½ cup)**
**calories: 138 | fat: 2g | protein: 8g | carbs: 23g | sugars: 4g | fiber: 7g | sodium: 0mg**

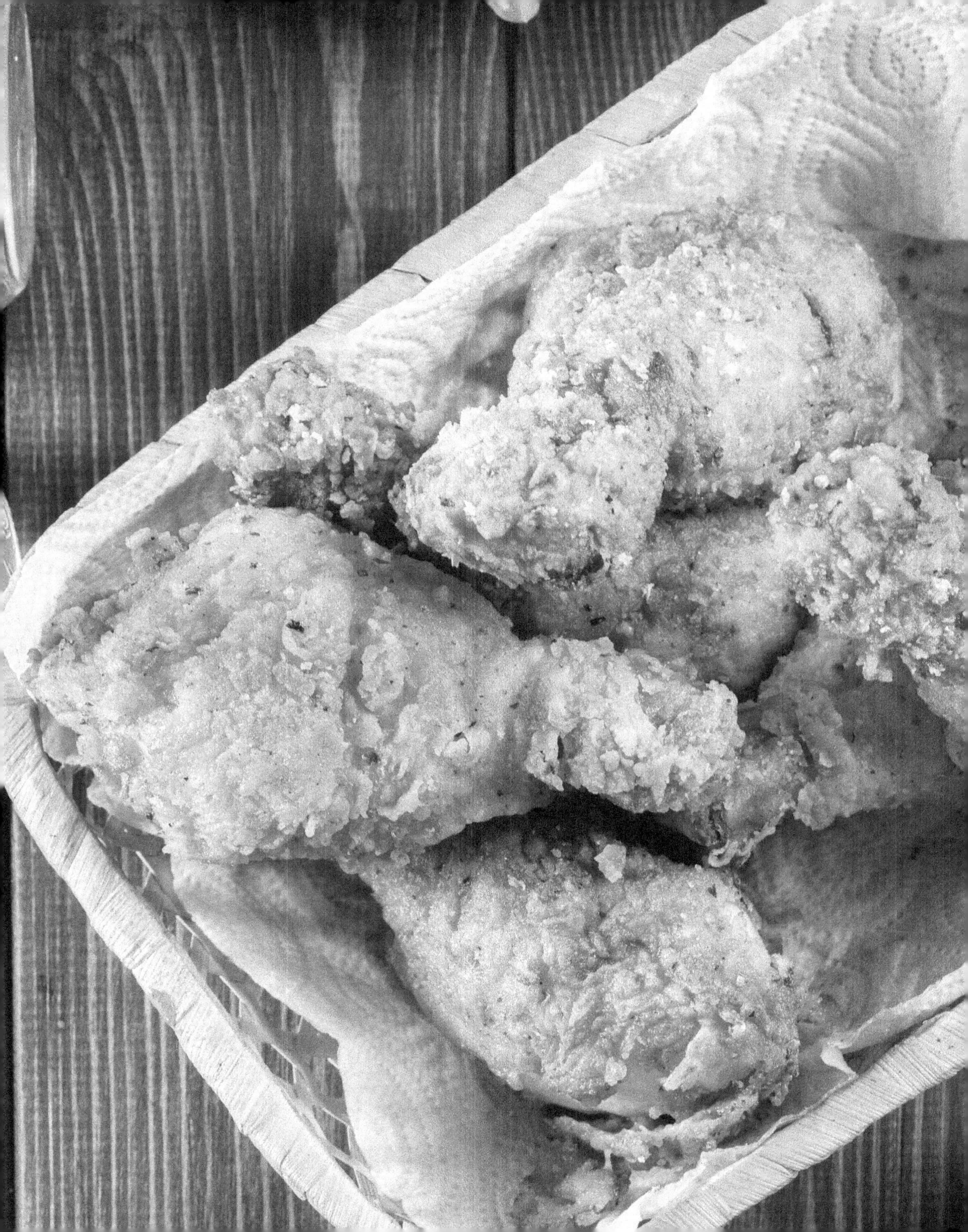

# Chapter 8 Poultry

94   **Shredded Buffalo Chicken**   79

95   **Buttery Lemon Chicken**   79

96   **Herbed Whole Turkey Breast**   80

97   **Garlic Galore Rotisserie Chicken**   80

98   **Greek Chicken**   81

99   **Chicken with Spiced Sesame Sauce**   81

100   **Chicken in Wine**   82

101   **Chicken Casablanca**   82

102   **Thai Yellow Curry with Chicken Meatballs**   82

103   **Sausage and Cauliflower "Grits"**   83

104   **Ground Turkey Tetrazzini**   84

105   **Szechuan-Style Chicken and Broccoli**   84

106   **Pulled BBQ Chicken and Texas-Style Cabbage Slaw**   85

107   **Chicken Reuben Bake**   86

108   **Mexican Turkey Tenderloin**   86

109   **Mild Chicken Curry with Coconut Milk**   86

110   **Smoky Whole Chicken**   87

111   **Chicken in Mushroom Gravy**   88

# Shredded Buffalo Chicken

**Prep time: 10 minutes | Cook time: 20 minutes | Serves 8**

2 tablespoons avocado oil

1 celery stalk, finely chopped

⅓ cup mild hot sauce (such as Frank's RedHot)

¼ teaspoon garlic powder

½ cup finely chopped onion

1 large carrot, chopped

½ tablespoon apple cider vinegar

2 bone-in, skin-on chicken breasts (about 2 pounds / 907 g)

1. Set the electric pressure cooker to the Sauté setting. When the pot is hot, pour in the avocado oil.
2. Sauté the onion, celery, and carrot for 3 to 5 minutes or until the onion begins to soften. Hit Cancel.
3. Stir in the hot sauce, vinegar, and garlic powder. Place the chicken breasts in the sauce, meat-side down.
4. Close and lock the lid of the pressure cooker. Set the valve to sealing.
5. Cook on high pressure for 20 minutes.
6. When cooking is complete, hit Cancel and quick release the pressure. Once the pin drops, unlock and remove the lid.
7. Using tongs, transfer the chicken breasts to a cutting board. When the chicken is cool enough to handle, remove the skin, shred the chicken and return it to the pot. Let the chicken soak in the sauce for at least 5 minutes.
8. Serve immediately.

**Per Serving (½ cup)**
calories: 139 | fat: 9g | protein: 12g | carbs: 2g | sugars: 1g | fiber: 1g | sodium: 295mg

# Buttery Lemon Chicken

**Prep time: 15 minutes | Cook time: 7 minutes | Serves 4**

2 tablespoons margarine

4 cloves garlic, minced

½ teaspoon pepper

1 teaspoon dried parsley, or 1 tablespoon chopped fresh parsley

2 pounds (907 g) boneless chicken breasts or thighs

½ cup low-sodium chicken broth

1 teaspoon salt

1 tablespoon water

1 medium onion, chopped

½ teaspoon paprika

⅓ cup lemon juice

1 to 2 tablespoons cornstarch

1. Set the Instant Pot to Sauté. When it is hot, add margarine to the inner pot and melt.
2. Add the onion, garlic, paprika, pepper, and parsley to melted margarine and sauté until onion starts to soften. Push onion to side of pot.
3. With the Instant Pot still at Sauté, add the chicken and sear on each side 3 to 5 minutes.
4. Mix broth, lemon juice, and salt together. Pour over chicken and stir to mix together.
5. Put on lid and set Instant Pot, move vent to sealing, and press Poultry. Set cook time for 7 minutes. Let depressurize naturally.
6. Remove chicken, leaving sauce in pot. Mix cornstarch in water and add to sauce. (Can start with 1 tablespoon cornstarch, and use second one if sauce isn't thick enough.)

**Per Serving**
calories: 350 | fat: 12g | protein: 52g | carbs: 6g | sugars: 1g | fiber: 0g | sodium: 658mg

# Herbed Whole Turkey Breast

**Prep time: 10 minutes | Cook time: 30 minutes | Serves 12**

3 tablespoons extra-virgin olive oil
1½ tablespoons herbes de Provence or poultry seasoning
2 teaspoons minced garlic
1 teaspoon lemon zest (from 1 small lemon)
1 tablespoon kosher salt
1½ teaspoons freshly ground black pepper
1 (6-pound / 2.7-kg) bone-in, skin-on whole turkey breast, rinsed and patted dry

1. In a small bowl, whisk together the olive oil, herbes de Provence, garlic, lemon zest, salt, and pepper.
2. Rub the outside of the turkey and under the skin with the olive oil mixture.
3. Pour 1 cup of water into the electric pressure cooker and insert a wire rack or trivet.
4. Place the turkey on the rack, skin-side up.
5. Close and lock the lid of the pressure cooker. Set the valve to sealing.
6. Cook on high pressure for 30 minutes.
7. When the cooking is complete, hit Cancel. Allow the pressure to release naturally for 20 minutes, then quick release any remaining pressure.
8. Once the pin drops, unlock and remove the lid.
9. Carefully transfer the turkey to a cutting board. Remove the skin, slice, and serve.

**Per Serving**
calories: 146 | fat: 9g | protein: 16g | carbs: 0g | sugars: 0g | fiber: 0g | sodium: 413mg

# Garlic Galore Rotisserie Chicken

**Prep time: 5 minutes | Cook time: 3 minutes | Serves 4**

3 pounds (1.4 kg) whole chicken
Salt, to taste
20 to 30 cloves fresh garlic, peeled and left whole
1 cup low-sodium chicken stock, broth, or water
2 tablespoons garlic powder
½ teaspoon basil
½ teaspoon chili powder

2 tablespoons olive oil, divided
Pepper, to taste

2 teaspoons onion powder
½ teaspoon cumin

1. Rub chicken with one tablespoon of the olive oil and sprinkle with salt and pepper.
2. Place the garlic cloves inside the chicken. Use butcher's twine to secure the legs.
3. Press the Sauté button on the Instant Pot, then add the rest of the olive oil to the inner pot.
4. When the pot is hot, place the chicken inside. You are just trying to sear it, so leave it for about 4 minutes on each side.
5. Remove the chicken and set aside. Place the trivet at the bottom of the inner pot and pour in the chicken stock.
6. Mix together the remaining seasonings and rub them all over the entire chicken.
7. Place the chicken back inside the inner pot, breast-side up, on top of the trivet and secure the lid to the sealing position.

8. Press the Manual button and use the "+/-" button to set it for 25 minutes.
9. When the timer beeps, allow the pressure to release naturally for 15 minutes. If the lid will not open at this point, quick release the remaining pressure and remove the chicken.
10. Let the chicken rest for 5 to 10 minutes before serving.

**Per Serving**
calories: 333 | fat: 23g | protein: 24g | carbs: 9g | sugars: 0g | fiber: 1g | sodium: 110mg

# Greek Chicken

**Prep time: 25 minutes | Cook time: 20 minutes | Serves 6**

**4 potatoes, unpeeled, quartered**
**2 pounds (907 g) chicken pieces, trimmed of skin and fat**
**2 large onions, quartered**
**3 teaspoons dried oregano**
**½ teaspoon pepper**
**1 cup water**

**1 whole bulb garlic, cloves minced**
**¾ teaspoons salt**
**1 tablespoon olive oil**

1. Place potatoes, chicken, onions, and garlic into the inner pot of the Instant Pot, then sprinkle with seasonings. Top with oil and water.
2. Secure the lid and make sure vent is set to sealing. Cook on Manual mode for 20 minutes.
3. When cook time is over, let the pressure release naturally for 5 minutes, then release the rest manually.

**Per Serving**
calories: 278 | fat: 6g | protein: 27g | carbs: 29g | sugars: 9g | fiber: 4g | sodium: 358mg

# Chicken with Spiced Sesame Sauce

**Prep time: 20 minutes | Cook time: 8 minutes | Serves 5**

**2 tablespoons tahini (sesame sauce)**
**1 tablespoon low-sodium soy sauce**
**1 teaspoon red wine vinegar**
**1 teaspoon shredded ginger root (Microplane works best)**
**2 pounds (907 g) chicken breast, chopped into 8 portions**

**¼ cup water**
**¼ cup chopped onion**
**2 teaspoons minced garlic**

1. Place first seven ingredients in bottom of the inner pot of the Instant Pot.
2. Add coarsely chopped chicken on top.
3. Secure the lid and make sure vent is at sealing. Set for 8 minutes using Manual setting. When cook time is up, let the pressure release naturally for 10 minutes, then perform a quick release.
4. Remove ingredients and shred chicken with fork. Combine with other ingredients in pot for a tasty sandwich filling or sauce.

**Per Serving**
calories: 215 | fat: 7g | protein: 35g | carbs: 2g | sugars: 0g | fiber: 0g | sodium: 178mg

# Chicken in Wine

**Prep time: 10 minutes | Cook time: 12 minutes | Serves 6**

2 pounds (907 g) chicken breasts, trimmed of skin and fat
1 (10¾-ounce / 305-g) can 98% fat-free, reduced-sodium cream of mushroom soup
1 (10¾-ounce / 305-g) can French onion soup       1 cup dry white wine or chicken broth

1.  Place the chicken into the Instant Pot.
2.  Combine soups and wine. Pour over chicken.
3.  Secure the lid and make sure vent is set to sealing. Cook on Manual mode for 12 minutes.
4.  When cook time is up, let the pressure release naturally for 5 minutes and then release the rest manually.

**Per Serving**
calories: 225 | fat: 5g | protein: 35g | carbs: 7g | sugars: 3g | fiber: 1g | sodium: 645mg

# Chicken Casablanca

**Prep time: 20 minutes | Cook time: 12 minutes | Serves 8**

2 large onions, sliced
3 garlic cloves, minced
3 pounds (1.4 kg) skinless chicken pieces
3 large carrots, diced
½ teaspoon ground cumin
½ teaspoon pepper
2 tablespoons raisins
3 small zucchini, sliced
1 (15-ounce / 425-g) can garbanzo beans, drained

1 teaspoon ground ginger
2 tablespoons canola oil, divided

2 large potatoes, unpeeled, diced
½ teaspoon salt
¼ teaspoon cinnamon
1 (14½-ounce / 411-g) can chopped tomatoes

2 tablespoons chopped parsley

1.  Using the Sauté function of the Instant Pot, cook the onions, ginger, and garlic in 1 tablespoon of the oil for 5 minutes, stirring constantly. Remove onions, ginger, and garlic from pot and set aside.
2.  Brown the chicken pieces with the remaining oil, then add the cooked onions, ginger and garlic back in as well as all of the remaining ingredients, except the parsley.
3.  Secure the lid and make sure vent is in the sealing position. Cook on Manual mode for 12 minutes.
4.  When cook time is up, let the pressure release naturally for 5 minutes and then release the rest of the pressure manually.

**Per Serving**
calories: 395 | fat: 10g | protein: 36g | carbs: 40g | sugars: 10g | fiber: 8g | sodium: 390mg

# Thai Yellow Curry with Chicken Meatballs

**Prep time: 5 minutes | Cook time: 30 minutes | Serves 4**

1 pound (454 g) 95 percent lean ground chicken
1 egg white
1 yellow onion, cut into 1-inch pieces
3 tablespoons yellow curry paste
8 ounces (227 g) carrots, halved lengthwise, then cut crosswise into 1-inch lengths (or quartered if very large)

⅓ cup gluten-free panko (Japanese bread crumbs)
1 tablespoon coconut oil
1 (14-ounce / 397-g) can light coconut milk
¾ cup water

8 ounces (227 g) zucchini, quartered lengthwise, then cut crosswise into 1-inch lengths (or cut into halves, then thirds if large)

8 ounces (227 g) cremini mushrooms, quartered    Fresh Thai basil leaves, for serving (optional)

Fresno or jalapeño chile, thinly sliced, for serving (optional)

1 lime, cut into wedges    Cooked cauliflower "rice", for serving

1. In a medium bowl, combine the chicken, panko, and egg white and mix until evenly combined. Set aside.
2. Select the Sauté setting on the Instant Pot and heat the oil for 2 minutes. Add the onion and sauté for 5 minutes, until it begins to soften and brown. Add ½ cup of the coconut milk and the curry paste and sauté for 1 minute more, until bubbling and fragrant. Press the Cancel button to turn off the pot, then stir in the water.
3. Using a 1½-tablespoon cookie scoop, shape and drop meatballs into the pot in a single layer.
4. Secure the lid and set the Pressure Release to Sealing. Select the Manual setting and set the cooking time for 5 minutes at high pressure. (The pot will take about 5 minutes to come up to pressure before the cooking program begins.)
5. When the cooking program ends, perform a quick pressure release by moving the Pressure Release to Venting, or let the pressure release naturally. Open the pot and stir in the carrots, zucchini, mushrooms, and remaining 1¼ cups coconut milk.
6. Press the Cancel button to reset the cooking program, then select the Sauté setting. Bring the curry to a simmer (this will take about 2 minutes), then let cook, uncovered, for about 8 minutes, until the carrots are fork-tender. Press the Cancel button to turn off the pot.
7. Ladle the curry into bowls. Serve piping hot, topped with basil leaves and chile slices, if desired, and the lime wedges and cauliflower "rice" on the side.

**Per Serving**
**calories: 349 | fat: 15g | protein: 30g | carbs: 34g | sugars: 8g | fiber: 5g | sodium: 529mg**

## Sausage and Cauliflower "Grits"

**Prep time: 7 minutes | Cook time: 20 minutes | Serves 4**

1 pound (454 g) frozen (uncooked) Italian-style chicken or turkey sausages

1 pound (454 g) frozen riced cauliflower, broken up

1 tablespoon extra-virgin olive oil    Freshly ground black pepper, to taste

⅓ cup shredded Parmesan cheese    Chopped fresh parsley, for garnish

1. Pour ½ cup of water into the electric pressure cooker and add the sausages.
2. Close and lock the lid of the pressure cooker. Set the valve to sealing.
3. Cook on high pressure for 15 minutes.
4. When the cooking is complete, hit Cancel and quick release the pressure.
5. Once the pin drops, unlock and remove the lid.
6. Using tongs, transfer the sausages to a cutting board and slice into 1-inch rounds. Pour the liquid from the pot into a measuring cup. Pour ½ cup of the liquid back into the pot; discard the rest.
7. In the electric pressure cooker, combine the sliced sausage, cauliflower, olive oil, and pepper. Close and lock the lid of the pressure cooker. Set the valve to sealing.
8. Cook on high pressure for 5 minutes.
9. When the cooking is complete, hit Cancel and quick release the pressure.
10. Once the pin drops, unlock and remove the lid.
11. Stir in the Parmesan, garnish with parsley, and serve immediately.

**Per Serving**
**calories: 263 | fat: 11g | protein: 30g | carbs: 11g | sugars: 4g | fiber: 3g | sodium: 660mg**

# Ground Turkey Tetrazzini



1 tablespoon extra-virgin olive oil

1 yellow onion, diced

½ teaspoon fine sea salt

1 pound (454 g) 93 percent lean ground turkey

6 ounces (170 g) whole-grain extra-broad egg-white pasta (such as No Yolks brand) or whole-wheat elbow pasta

1½ cups frozen green peas, thawed

3 (¾-ounce / 21-g) wedges Laughing Cow creamy light Swiss cheese, or 2 tablespoons Neufchâtel cheese, at room temperature

1 tablespoon chopped fresh flat-leaf parsley

2 garlic cloves, minced

8 ounces (227 g) cremini or button mushrooms, sliced

¼ teaspoon freshly ground black pepper

1 teaspoon poultry seasoning

2 cups low-sodium chicken broth

3 cups baby spinach

⅓ cup grated Parmesan cheese

1. Select the Sauté setting on the Instant Pot and heat the oil and garlic for 2 minutes, until the garlic is bubbling but not browned. Add the onion, mushrooms, salt, and pepper and sauté for about 5 minutes, until the mushrooms have wilted and begun to give up their liquid. Add the turkey and poultry seasoning and sauté, using a wooden spoon or spatula to break up the meat as it cooks, for about 4 minutes more, until cooked through and no streaks of pink remain.
2. Stir in the pasta. Pour in the broth and use the spoon or spatula to nudge the pasta into the liquid as much as possible. It's fine if some pieces are not completely submerged.
3. Secure the lid and set the Pressure Release to Sealing. Press the Cancel button to reset the cooking program, then select the Manual setting and set the cooking time for 5 minutes at high pressure. (The pot will take about 5 minutes to come up to pressure before the cooking program begins.)
4. When the cooking program ends, let the pressure release naturally for 5 minutes, then move the Pressure Release to Venting to release any remaining steam. Open the pot and stir in the peas, spinach, Laughing Cow cheese, and Parmesan. Let stand for 2 minutes, then stir the mixture once more.
5. Ladle into bowls or onto plates and sprinkle with the parsley. Serve right away.

**Per Serving**

calories: 321 | fat: 11g | protein: 26g | carbs: 35g | sugars: 4g | fiber: 5g | sodium: 488mg

# Szechuan-Style Chicken and Broccoli



1 tablespoon canola oil

2 whole boneless, skinless chicken breasts, cut into 1-inch cubes

2 cups broccoli florets

½ cup picante sauce

2 tablespoons light soy sauce

2 teaspoons quick-cooking tapioca

2 garlic cloves, minced

1 medium red bell pepper, sliced

½ cup low-sodium chicken stock

½ teaspoon sugar

1 medium onion, chopped

½ teaspoon ground ginger

1. Set the Instant Pot to Sauté and add the oil and chicken. Sauté until lightly browned. Press Cancel.
2. Add in the broccoli and bell pepper. In a small bowl, mix together the remaining ingredients, then pour over the contents of the Instant Pot and stir.

3. Secure the lid and make sure vent is at sealing. Cook in Manual mode for 12 minutes.
4. When cooking time is over, let the pressure release naturally for 5 minutes, then release the rest manually.

**Per Serving**
calories: 217 | fat: 7g | protein: 27g | carbs: 11g | sugars: 5g | fiber: 2g | sodium: 425mg

# Pulled BBQ Chicken and Texas-Style Cabbage Slaw

**Prep time: 5 minutes | Cook time: 20 minutes | Serves 6**

**Chicken:**
1 cup water
3 garlic cloves, peeled
2 pounds (907 g) boneless, skinless chicken thighs
**Cabbage Slaw:**
½ head red or green cabbage, thinly sliced
1 red bell pepper, seeded and thinly sliced
2 jalapeño chiles, seeded and cut into narrow strips
2 carrots, julienned
½ cup chopped fresh cilantro
3 tablespoons extra-virgin olive oil
¼ teaspoon fine sea salt

¼ teaspoon fine sea salt
2 bay leaves

1 large Fuji or Gala apple, julienned
3 tablespoons fresh lime juice
½ teaspoon ground cumin

¾ cup low-sugar or unsweetened barbecue sauce
Cornbread, for serving

1. To make the chicken: Combine the water, salt, garlic, bay leaves, and chicken thighs in the Instant Pot, arranging the chicken in a single layer.
2. Secure the lid and set the Pressure Release to Sealing. Select the Poultry or Manual setting and set the cooking time for 10 minutes at high pressure. (The pot will take about 10 minutes to come up to pressure before the cooking program begins.)
3. To make the slaw: While the chicken is cooking, in a large bowl, combine the cabbage, bell pepper, jalapeños, carrots, apple, cilantro, lime juice, oil, cumin, and salt and toss together until the vegetables and apples are evenly coated.
4. When the cooking program ends, perform a quick pressure release by moving the Pressure Release to Venting, or let the pressure release naturally. Open the pot and, using tongs, transfer the chicken to a cutting board. Using two forks, shred the chicken into bite-size pieces. Wearing heat-resistant mitts, lift out the inner pot and discard the cooking liquid. Return the inner pot to the housing.
5. Return the chicken to the pot and stir in the barbecue sauce. You can serve it right away or heat it for a minute or two on the Sauté setting, then return the pot to its Keep Warm setting until ready to serve.
6. Divide the chicken and slaw evenly among six plates. Serve with wedges of cornbread on the side.

**Per Serving (without cornbread)**
calories: 320 | fat: 14g | protein: 32g | carbs: 18g | sugars: 7g | fiber: 4g | sodium: 386mg

# Chicken Reuben Bake

**Prep time: 10 minutes | Cook time: 6 to 8 hours | Serves 6**

4 boneless, skinless chicken-breast halves

¼ cup water

1 (1-pound / 454-g) bag sauerkraut, drained and rinsed

4 to 5 (1 ounce / 28 g each) slices Swiss cheese

¾ cup fat-free Thousand Island salad dressing

2 tablespoons chopped fresh parsley

1. Place chicken and water in inner pot of the Instant Pot along with ¼ cup water. Layer sauerkraut over chicken. Add cheese. Top with salad dressing. Sprinkle with parsley.
2. Secure the lid and cook on the Slow Cook setting on low 6 to 8 hours.

**Per Serving**

calories: 217 | fat: 5g | protein: 28g | carbs: 13g | sugars: 6g | fiber: 2g | sodium: 693mg

# Mexican Turkey Tenderloin

**Prep time: 5 minutes | Cook time: 8 minutes | Serves 6**

1 cup bottled salsa

1 teaspoon chili powder

½ teaspoon ground cumin

¼ teaspoon dried oregano

1½ pounds (680 g) unseasoned turkey tenderloin or boneless turkey breast, cut into 6 pieces

Freshly ground black pepper, to taste

½ cup shredded Monterey Jack cheese or Mexican cheese blend

1. In a small bowl or measuring cup, combine the salsa, chili powder, cumin, and oregano. Pour half of the mixture into the electric pressure cooker.
2. Nestle the turkey into the sauce. Grind some pepper onto each piece of turkey. Pour the remaining salsa mixture on top.
3. Close and lock the lid of the pressure cooker. Set the valve to sealing.
4. Cook on high pressure for 8 minutes.
5. When the cooking is complete, hit Cancel. Allow the pressure to release naturally for 10 minutes, then quick release any remaining pressure.
6. Once the pin drops, unlock and remove the lid.
7. Sprinkle the cheese on top, and put the lid back on for a few minutes to let the cheese melt.
8. Serve immediately.

**Per Serving**

calories: 168 | fat: 5g | protein: 28g | carbs: 3g | sugars: 2g | fiber: 1g | sodium: 559mg

# Mild Chicken Curry with Coconut Milk

**Prep time: 10 minutes | Cook time: 14 minutes | Serves 4 to 6**

1 large onion, diced

6 cloves garlic, crushed

¼ cup coconut oil

½ teaspoon black pepper

½ teaspoon turmeric

½ teaspoon paprika

¼ teaspoon cinnamon

¼ teaspoon cloves

¼ teaspoon cumin

¼ teaspoon ginger

½ teaspoon salt

1 tablespoon curry powder (more if you like more flavor)

½ teaspoon chili powder

1 (24-ounce / 680-g) can low-sodium diced or crushed tomatoes

1 (13½-ounce / 383-g) can light coconut milk

4 pounds (1.8 kg) boneless skinless chicken breasts, cut into chunks

1. Sauté onion and garlic in the coconut oil, either with Sauté setting in the inner pot of the Instant Pot or on stove top, then add to pot.
2. Combine spices in a small bowl, then add to the inner pot.
3. Add tomatoes and coconut milk and stir.
4. Add chicken, and stir to coat the pieces with the sauce.
5. Secure the lid and make sure vent is at sealing. Set to Manual mode for 14 minutes.
6. Let pressure release naturally (if you're crunched for time, you can do a quick release).
7. Serve with your favorite sides, and enjoy!

**Per Serving**
calories: 535 | fat: 21g | protein: 71g | carbs: 10g | sugars: 5g | fiber: 2g | sodium: 315mg

## Smoky Whole Chicken

**Prep time: 20 minutes | Cook time: 21 minutes | Serves 6**

2 tablespoons extra-virgin olive oil

1 tablespoon kosher salt

1½ teaspoons smoked paprika

1 teaspoon freshly ground black pepper

½ teaspoon herbes de Provence

¼ teaspoon cayenne pepper

1 (3½-pound / 1.6-kg) whole chicken, rinsed and patted dry, giblets removed

1 large lemon, halved

6 garlic cloves, peeled and crushed with the flat side of a knife

1 large onion, cut into 8 wedges, divided

1 cup low-sodium store-bought chicken broth or water

2 large carrots, each cut into 4 pieces

2 celery stalks, each cut into 4 pieces

1. In a small bowl, combine the olive oil, salt, paprika, pepper, herbes de Provence, and cayenne.
2. Place the chicken on a cutting board and rub the olive oil mixture under the skin and all over the outside. Stuff the cavity with the lemon halves, garlic cloves, and 3 to 4 wedges of onion.
3. Pour the broth into the electric pressure cooker. Add the remaining onion wedges, carrots, and celery. Insert a wire rack or trivet on top of the vegetables.
4. Place the chicken, breast-side up, on the rack.
5. Close and lock the lid of the pressure cooker. Set the valve to sealing.
6. Cook on high pressure for 21 minutes.
7. When the cooking is complete, hit Cancel and allow the pressure to release naturally for 15 minutes, then quick release any remaining pressure.
8. Once the pin drops, unlock and remove the lid.
9. Carefully remove the chicken to a clean cutting board. Remove the skin and cut the chicken into pieces or shred/chop the meat, and serve.

**Per Serving**
calories: 215 | fat: 9g | protein: 25g | carbs: 5g | sugars: 2g | fiber: 1g | sodium: 847mg

# Chicken in Mushroom Gravy

**Prep time: 10 minutes | Cook time: 10 minutes | Serves 6**

6 (5 ounces / 142 g each) boneless, skinless chicken-breast halves
Salt and pepper, to taste
¼ cup dry white wine or low-sodium chicken broth
1 (10¾-ounce / 305-g) can 98% fat-free, reduced-sodium cream of mushroom soup
4 ounces (113 g) sliced mushrooms

1. Place chicken in the inner pot of the Instant Pot. Season with salt and pepper.
2. Combine wine and soup in a bowl, then pour over the chicken. Top with the mushrooms.
3. Secure the lid and make sure the vent is set to sealing. Set on Manual mode for 10 minutes.
4. When cooking time is up, let the pressure release naturally.

**Per Serving**
calories: 204 | fat: 4g | protein: 34g | carbs: 6g | sugars: 1g | fiber: 1g | sodium: 320mg

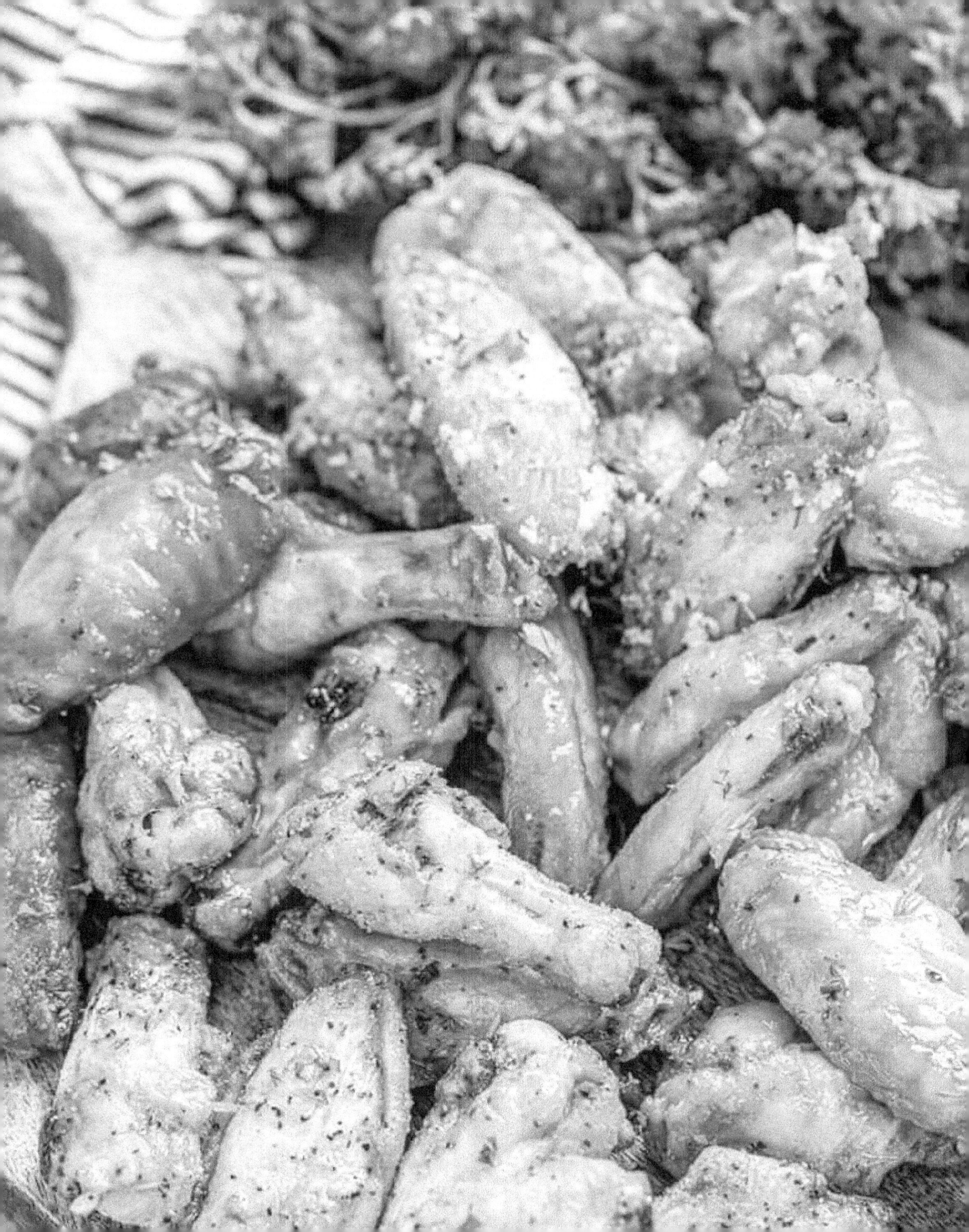

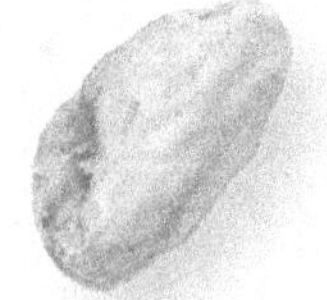

112    Carnitas Burrito Bowls    91

113    Machaca Beef    92

114    Beef Roast with Mushroom Barley    92

115    Pork Chops Pomodoro    92

116    Beef Burgundy    93

117    Pork Carnitas    94

118    Rosemary Lamb Chops    94

119    5-Ingredient Mexican Lasagna    95

120    Bavarian Beef    96

121    Pot Roast with Gravy and Vegetables    96

122    Steak Stroganoff    97

123    Asian Pepper Steak    97

124    Pork Butt Roast    98

125    Spicy Beef Stew with Butternut Squash    98

126    BBQ Ribs and Broccoli Slaw    99

127    "Smothered" Steak    100

# Carnitas Burrito Bowls



**Carnitas:**

1 tablespoon chili powder

1 teaspoon ground coriander

½ cup water

½ teaspoon garlic powder

1 teaspoon fine sea salt

¼ cup fresh lime juice

1 (2-pound / 907-g) boneless pork shoulder butt roast, cut into 2-inch cubes

**Rice and Beans:**

1 cup Minute brand brown rice

1½ cups drained cooked black beans, or 1 (15-ounce / 425-g) can black beans, rinsed and drained

**Pico de Gallo:**

8 ounces (227 g) tomatoes, diced

1 jalapeño chile, seeded and finely diced

1 teaspoon fresh lime juice

½ small yellow onion, diced

1 tablespoon chopped fresh cilantro

Pinch of fine sea salt

¼ cup sliced green onions, white and green parts

2 tablespoons chopped fresh cilantro

3 hearts romaine lettuce, cut into ¼-inch-wide ribbons  2 large avocados, pitted, peeled, and sliced

Hot sauce (such as Cholula or Tapatío), for serving

1. To make the carnitas: In a small bowl, combine the chili powder, garlic powder, coriander, and salt and mix well.
2. Pour the water and lime juice into the Instant Pot. Add the pork, arranging the pieces in a single layer. Sprinkle the chili powder mixture evenly over the pork.
3. Secure the lid and set the Pressure Release to Sealing. Select the Meat/Stew setting and set the cooking time for 30 minutes at high pressure. (The pot will take about 10 minutes to come up to pressure before the cooking program begins.)
4. When the cooking program ends, let the pressure release naturally for at least 15 minutes, then move the Pressure Release to Venting to release any remaining steam. Open the pot and, using tongs, transfer the pork to a plate or cutting board.
5. While the pressure is releasing, preheat the oven to 400ºF (205ºC).
6. Wearing heat-resistant mitts, lift out the inner pot and pour the cooking liquid into a fat separator. Pour the defatted cooking liquid into a liquid measuring cup and discard the fat. (Alternatively, use a ladle or large spoon to skim the fat off the surface of the liquid.) Add water as needed to the cooking liquid to total 1 cup (you may have enough without adding water).
7. To make the rice and beans: Pour the 1 cup cooking liquid into the Instant Pot and add the rice, making sure it is in an even layer. Place a tall steam rack into the pot. Add the black beans to a 1½-quart stainless-steel bowl and place the bowl on top of the rack. (The bowl should not touch the lid once the pot is closed.)
8. Secure the lid and set the Pressure Release to Sealing. Press the Cancel button to reset the cooking program, then select the Manual setting and set the cooking time for 15 minutes at high pressure. (The pot will take about 5 minutes to come to pressure before the cooking program begins.)
9. While the rice and beans are cooking, using two forks, shred the meat into bite-size pieces. Transfer the pork to a sheet pan, spreading it out in an even layer. Place in the oven for 20 minutes, until crispy and browned.
10. To make the pico de gallo: While the carnitas, rice, and beans are cooking, in a medium bowl, combine the tomatoes, onion, jalapeño, cilantro, lime juice, and salt and mix well. Set aside.
11. When the cooking program ends, let the pressure release naturally for 5 minutes, then move the Pressure Release to Venting to release any remaining steam. Open the pot and, wearing heat-resistant mitts, remove the bowl of beans and then the steam rack from the pot. Then remove the inner pot. Add the green onions and cilantro to the rice and, using a fork, fluff the rice and mix in the green onions and cilantro.
12. Divide the rice, beans, carnitas, pico de gallo, lettuce, and avocados evenly among six bowls. Serve warm, with the hot sauce on the side.

**Per Serving**

calories: 447 | fat: 20g | protein: 31g | carbs: 35g | sugars: 4g | fiber: 9g | sodium: 653mg

# Machaca Beef



1½ pounds (680 g) beef roast
1 (4-ounce / 113-g) can chopped green chilies
1½ teaspoons dry mustard
1 teaspoon seasoning salt
1 cup water

1 large onion, sliced
2 beef bouillon cubes
½ teaspoon garlic powder
½ teaspoon pepper
1 cup salsa

1.  Combine all ingredients except salsa in the Instant Pot inner pot.
2.  Secure the lid and make sure the vent is set to sealing. Press the Slow Cook button and set on low for 12 hours, or until beef is tender. Drain and reserve liquid.
3.  Shred beef using two forks to pull it apart.
4.  Combine beef, salsa, and enough of the reserved liquid to make desired consistency.
5.  Use this filling for burritos, chalupas, quesadillas, or tacos.

**Per Serving**
calories: 69 | fat: 2g | protein: 9g | carbs: 3g | sugars: 2g | fiber: 1g | sodium: 392mg

# Beef Roast with Mushroom Barley

Prep time: 20 minutes | Cook time: 1 hour 15 minutes | Serves 6

1 tablespoon olive oil
1 cup pearl barley (not quick-cook)
1 (6½-ounce / 184-g) can mushrooms, undrained
1 teaspoon minced garlic
¼ teaspoon black pepper

2 pounds (907 g) beef chuck roast, visible fat removed
½ cup onion, diced

1 teaspoon Italian seasoning
1¾ cups beef broth

1.  Press the Sauté button on the Instant Pot and pour the oil in to warm up. Brown the roast for about 5 minutes on each side. Press Cancel.
2.  Add the rest of the ingredients to the Instant Pot, then secure the lid, making sure the vent is set to sealing.
3.  Press the Manual button and set the time for 1 hour and 15 minutes.
4.  When cook time is up, let the pressure release naturally for 15 minutes, then perform a quick release.

**Per Serving**
calories: 353 | fat: 12g | protein: 37g | carbs: 25g | sugars: 1g | fiber: 6g | sodium: 354mg

# Pork Chops Pomodoro

Prep time: 5 minutes | Cook time: 30 minutes | Serves 6

2 pounds (907 g) boneless pork loin chops, each about 5⅓ ounces (150 g) and ½ inch thick
¾ teaspoon fine sea salt
2 tablespoons extra-virgin olive oil
½ cup low-sodium chicken broth or vegetable broth
½ teaspoon Italian seasoning

½ teaspoon freshly ground black pepper
2 garlic cloves, chopped

1 tablespoon capers, drained

2 cups cherry tomatoes

2 tablespoons chopped fresh basil or flat-leaf parsley

Spiralized zucchini noodles, cooked cauliflower "rice," or cooked whole-grain pasta for serving

Lemon wedges, for serving

1. Pat the pork chops dry with paper towels, then season them all over with the salt and pepper.
2. Select the Sauté setting on the Instant Pot and heat 1 tablespoon of the oil for 2 minutes. Swirl the oil to coat the bottom of the pot. Using tongs, add half of the pork chops in a single layer and sear for about 3 minutes, until lightly browned on the first side. Flip the chops and sear for about 3 minutes more, until lightly browned on the second side. Transfer the chops to a plate. Repeat with the remaining 1 tablespoon oil and pork chops.
3. Add the garlic to the pot and sauté for about 1 minute, until bubbling but not browned. Stir in the broth, Italian seasoning, and capers, using a wooden spoon to nudge any browned bits from the bottom of the pot and working quickly so not too much liquid evaporates. Using the tongs, transfer the pork chops to the pot. Add the tomatoes in an even layer on top of the chops.
4. Secure the lid and set the Pressure Release to Sealing. Press the Cancel button to reset the cooking program, then select the Manual setting and set the cooking time for 10 minutes at high pressure. (The pot will take about 5 minutes to come up to pressure before the cooking program begins.)
5. When the cooking program ends, let the pressure release naturally for at least 10 minutes, then move the Pressure Release to Venting to release any remaining steam. Open the pot and, using the tongs, transfer the pork chops to a serving dish.
6. Spoon the tomatoes and some of the cooking liquid on top of the pork chops. Sprinkle with the basil and serve right away, with zucchini noodles and lemon wedges on the side.

**Per Serving**

calories: 265 | fat: 13g | protein: 31g | carbs: 3g | sugars: 2g | fiber: 1g | sodium: 460mg

# Beef Burgundy

**Prep time: 30 minutes | Cook time: 30 minutes | Serves 6**

2 tablespoons olive oil

2½ tablespoons flour

½ pound (227 g) fresh mushrooms, sliced

¼ teaspoon dried marjoram

⅛ teaspoon pepper

1½ cups burgundy

2 pounds (907 g) stewing meat, cubed, trimmed of fat

5 medium onions, thinly sliced

1 teaspoon salt

¼ teaspoon dried thyme

¾ cup beef broth

1. Press Sauté on the Instant pot and add in the olive oil.
2. Dredge meat in flour, then brown in batches in the Instant Pot. Set aside the meat. Sauté the onions and mushrooms in the remaining oil and drippings for about 3 to 4 minutes, then add the meat back in. Press Cancel.
3. Add the salt, marjoram, thyme, pepper, broth, and wine to the Instant Pot.
4. Secure the lid and make sure the vent is set to sealing. Press the Manual button and set to 30 minutes.
5. When cook time is up, let the pressure release naturally for 15 minutes, then perform a quick release.
6. Serve over cooked noodles.

**Per Serving**

calories: 358 | fat: 11g | protein: 37g | carbs: 15g | sugars: 5g | fiber: 2g | sodium: 472mg

# Pork Carnitas



1 teaspoon kosher salt

2 teaspoons chili powder

2 teaspoons dried oregano

½ teaspoon freshly ground black pepper

1 (2½-pound / 1.1-kg) pork sirloin roast or boneless pork butt, cut into 1½-inch cubes

2 tablespoons avocado oil, divided

3 garlic cloves, minced

Juice and zest of 1 large orange

Juice and zest of 1 medium lime

6-inch gluten-free corn tortillas, warmed, for serving (optional)

Chopped avocado, for serving (optional)

Salsa verde, for serving (optional)

Shredded Cheddar cheese, for serving (optional)

1.  In a large bowl or gallon-size zip-top bag, combine the salt, chili powder, oregano, and pepper. Add the pork cubes and toss to coat.
2.  Set the electric pressure cooker to the Sauté/More setting. When the pot is hot, pour in 1 tablespoon of avocado oil.
3.  Add half of the pork to the pot and sear until the pork is browned on all sides, about 5 minutes. Transfer the pork to a plate, add the remaining 1 tablespoon of avocado oil to the pot, and sear the remaining pork. Hit Cancel.
4.  Return all of the pork to the pot and add the garlic, orange zest and juice, and lime zest and juice to the pot.
5.  Close and lock the lid of the pressure cooker. Set the valve to sealing.
6.  Cook on high pressure for 20 minutes.
7.  When the cooking is complete, hit Cancel. Allow the pressure to release naturally for 15 minutes then quick release any remaining pressure.
8.  Once the pin drops, unlock and remove the lid.
9.  Using two forks, shred the meat right in the pot.
10. (Optional) For more authentic carnitas, spread the shredded meat on a broiler-safe sheet pan. Preheat the broiler with the rack 6 inches from the heating element. Broil the pork for about 5 minutes or until it begins to crisp. (Watch carefully so you don't let the pork burn.)
11. Place the pork in a serving bowl. Top with some of the juices from the pot. Serve with tortillas, avocado, salsa, and Cheddar cheese (if using).

**Per Serving**

calories: 150 | fat: 5g | protein: 22g | carbs: 3g | sugars: 1g | fiber: 1g | sodium: 245mg

# Rosemary Lamb Chops



1½ pounds (680 g) lamb chops (4 small chops)

1 teaspoon kosher salt

Leaves from 1 (6-inch) rosemary sprig

2 tablespoons avocado oil

1 shallot, peeled and cut in quarters

1 tablespoon tomato paste

1 cup beef broth

1.  Place the lamb chops on a cutting board. Press the salt and rosemary leaves into both sides of the chops. Let rest at room temperature for 15 to 30 minutes.

2.  Set the electric pressure cooker to Sauté/More setting. When hot, add the avocado oil.
3.  Brown the lamb chops, about 2 minutes per side. (If they don't all fit in a single layer, brown them in batches.)
4.  Transfer the chops to a plate. In the pot, combine the shallot, tomato paste, and broth. Cook for about a minute, scraping up the brown bits from the bottom. Hit Cancel.
5.  Add the chops and any accumulated juices back to the pot.
6.  Close and lock the lid of the pressure cooker. Set the valve to sealing.
7.  Cook on high pressure for 2 minutes.
8.  When the cooking is complete, hit Cancel and quick release the pressure.
9.  Once the pin drops, unlock and remove the lid.
10.  Place the lamb chops on plates and serve immediately.

**Per Serving (1 lamb chop)**
calories: 233 | fat: 18g | protein: 15g | carbs: 1g | sugars: 1g | fiber: 0g | sodium: 450mg

# 5-Ingredient Mexican Lasagna

**Prep time: 15 minutes | Cook time: 15 minutes | Serves 4**

**Nonstick cooking spray**
**½ (15-ounce / 425-g) can light red kidney beans, rinsed and drained**
**4 (6-inch) gluten-free corn tortillas**
**1½ cups cooked shredded beef, pork, or chicken**
**1⅓ cups salsa**
**1⅓ cups shredded Mexican cheese blend**

1.  Spray a 6-inch springform pan with nonstick spray. Wrap the bottom in foil.
2.  In a medium bowl, mash the beans with a fork.
3.  Place 1 tortilla in the bottom of the pan. Add about ⅓ of the beans, ½ cup of meat, ⅓ cup of salsa, and ⅓ cup of cheese. Press down. Repeat for 2 more layers. Add the remaining tortilla and press down. Top with the remaining salsa and cheese. There are no beans or meat on the top layer.
4.  Tear off a piece of foil big enough to cover the pan, and spray it with nonstick spray. Line the pan with the foil, sprayed-side down.
5.  Pour 1 cup of water into the electric pressure cooker.
6.  Place the pan on the wire rack and carefully lower it into the pot. Close and lock the lid of the pressure cooker. Set the valve to sealing.
7.  Cook on high pressure for 15 minutes.
8.  When the cooking is complete, hit Cancel. Allow the pressure to release naturally for 10 minutes, then quick release any remaining pressure.
9.  Once the pin drops, unlock and remove the lid.
10.  Using the handles of the wire rack, carefully remove the pan from the pot. Let the lasagna sit for 5 minutes. Carefully remove the ring.
11.  Slice into quarters and serve.

**Per Serving**
calories: 395 | fat: 16g | protein: 30g | carbs: 34g | sugars: 5g | fiber: 9g | sodium: 1140mg

# Bavarian Beef

**Prep time: 35 minutes | Cook time: 1 hour 15 minutes | Serves 8**

1 tablespoon canola oil
3 pounds (1.4 kg) boneless beef chuck roast, trimmed of fat

| | |
|---|---|
| 3 cups sliced carrots | 3 cups sliced onions |
| 2 large kosher dill pickles, chopped | 1 cup sliced celery |
| ½ cup dry red wine or beef broth | ⅓ cup German-style mustard |
| 2 teaspoons coarsely ground black pepper | 2 bay leaves |
| ¼ teaspoon ground cloves | 1 cup water |

⅓ cup flour

1. Press Sauté on the Instant Pot and add in the oil. Brown roast on both sides for about 5 minutes. Press Cancel.
2. Add all of the remaining ingredients, except for the flour, to the Instant Pot.
3. Secure the lid and make sure the vent is set to sealing. Press Manual and set the time to 1 hour and 15 minutes. Let the pressure release naturally.
4. Remove meat and vegetables to large platter. Cover to keep warm.
5. Remove 1 cup of the liquid from the Instant Pot and mix with the flour. Press Sauté on the Instant Pot and add the flour/broth mixture back in, whisking. Cook until the broth is smooth and thickened.
6. Serve over noodles or spaetzle.

**Per Serving**
calories: 251 | fat: 8g | protein: 26g | carbs: 17g | sugars: 7g | fiber: 4g | sodium: 525mg

# Pot Roast with Gravy and Vegetables

**Prep time: 30 minutes | Cook time: 1 hour 15 minutes | Serves 6**

1 tablespoon olive oil
3 to 4 pounds (1.4 to 1.8 kg) bottom round, rump, or arm roast, trimmed of fat

| | |
|---|---|
| ¼ teaspoon salt | 2 to 3 teaspoons pepper |
| 2 tablespoons flour | 1 cup cold water |

1 teaspoon Kitchen Bouquet, or gravy browning seasoning sauce

| | |
|---|---|
| 1 garlic clove, minced | 2 medium onions, cut in wedges |

4 medium potatoes, cubed, unpeeled
2 carrots, quartered
1 green bell pepper, sliced

1. Press the Sauté button on the Instant Pot and pour the oil inside, letting it heat up. Sprinkle each side of the roast with salt and pepper, then brown it for 5 minutes on each side inside the pot.
2. Mix together the flour, water and Kitchen Bouquet and spread over roast.
3. Add garlic, onions, potatoes, carrots, and green pepper.
4. Secure the lid and make sure the vent is set to sealing. Press Manual and set the Instant Pot for 1 hour and 15 minutes.
5. When cook time is up, let the pressure release naturally.

**Per Serving**
calories: 551 | fat: 30g | protein: 49g | carbs: 19g | sugars: 2g | fiber: 3g | sodium: 256mg

# Steak Stroganoff



**Prep time: 15 minutes | Cook time: 30 minutes | Serves 6**

1 tablespoon olive oil
2 tablespoons flour
½ teaspoon garlic powder
½ teaspoon pepper
¼ teaspoon paprika
1¾ pounds (794 g) boneless beef round steak, trimmed of fat, cut into 1½ × ½-inch strips
1 (10¾-ounce / 305-g) can reduced-sodium, 98% fat-free cream of mushroom soup
½ cup water
1 envelope sodium-free dried onion soup mix
1 (9-ounce / 255-g) jar sliced mushrooms, drained
½ cup fat-free sour cream
1 tablespoon minced fresh parsley

1. Place the oil in the Instant Pot and press Sauté.
2. Combine flour, garlic powder, pepper, and paprika in a small bowl. Stir the steak pieces through the flour mixture until they are evenly coated.
3. Lightly brown the steak pieces in the oil in the Instant Pot, about 2 minutes each side. Press Cancel when done.
4. Stir the mushroom soup, water, and onion soup mix then pour over the steak.
5. Secure the lid and set the vent to sealing. Press the Manual button and set for 15 minutes.
6. When cook time is up, let the pressure release naturally for 15 minutes, then release the rest manually.
7. Remove the lid and press Cancel then Sauté. Stir in mushrooms, sour cream, and parsley. Let the sauce come to a boil and cook for about 10 to 15 minutes.

**Per Serving**
calories: 248 | fat: 6g | protein: 33g | carbs: 12g | sugars: 2g | fiber: 2g | sodium: 563mg

# Asian Pepper Steak

**Prep time: 20 minutes | Cook time: 6 to 8 hours | Serves 6**

1 pound (454 g) round steak, sliced thin, trimmed of fat
3 tablespoons light soy sauce
1 garlic clove, minced
1 (4-ounce / 113-g) can mushrooms, drained, or 1 cup sliced fresh mushrooms
1 medium onion, thinly sliced
½ teaspoon ground ginger
1 medium green pepper, thinly sliced
½ teaspoon crushed red pepper

1. Combine all ingredients in the inner pot of the Instant Pot.
2. Secure the lid and press Slow Cook on low 6 to 8 hours.
3. Serve as steak sandwiches topped with provolone cheese, or over rice.

**Per Serving**
calories: 122 | fat: 4g | protein: 16g | carbs: 6g | sugars: 3g | fiber: 2g | sodium: 368mg

# Pork Butt Roast

**Prep time: 10 minutes | Cook time: 9 minutes | Serves 6 to 8**

3 to 4 pounds (1.4 to 1.8 kg) pork butt roast
2 to 3 tablespoons of your favorite rub
2 cups water

1.  Place pork in the inner pot of the Instant Pot.
2.  Sprinkle in the rub all over the roast and add the water, being careful not to wash off the rub.
3.  Secure the lid and set the vent to sealing. Cook for 9 minutes on the Manual setting.
4.  Let the pressure release naturally.

**Per Serving**
calories: 598 | fat: 40g | protein: 57g | carbs: 0g | sugars: 0g | fiber: 0g | sodium: 152mg

# Spicy Beef Stew with Butternut Squash

**Prep time: 15 minutes | Cook time: 30 minutes | Serves 8**

1½ tablespoons smoked paprika
2 teaspoons ground cinnamon
1½ teaspoons kosher salt
1 teaspoon ground ginger
1 teaspoon red pepper flakes
½ teaspoon freshly ground black pepper
2 pounds (907 g) beef shoulder roast, cut into 1-inch cubes
2 tablespoons avocado oil, divided
1 cup low-sodium beef or vegetable broth
1 medium red onion, cut into wedges
8 garlic cloves, minced
1 (28-ounce / 794-g) carton or can no-salt-added diced tomatoes
2 pounds (907 g) butternut squash, peeled and cut into 1-inch pieces
Chopped fresh cilantro or parsley, for serving

1.  In a zip-top bag or medium bowl, combine the paprika, cinnamon, salt, ginger, red pepper, and black pepper. Add the beef and toss to coat.
2.  Set the electric pressure cooker to the Sauté setting. When the pot is hot, pour in 1 tablespoon of avocado oil.
3.  Add half of the beef to the pot and cook, stirring occasionally, for 3 to 5 minutes or until the beef is no longer pink. Transfer it to a plate, then add the remaining 1 tablespoon of avocado oil and brown the remaining beef. Transfer to the plate. Hit Cancel.
4.  Stir in the broth and scrape up any brown bits from the bottom of the pot. Return the beef to the pot and add the onion, garlic, tomatoes and their juices, and squash. Stir well.
5.  Close and lock lid of pressure cooker. Set the valve to sealing.
6.  Cook on high pressure for 30 minutes.
7.  When cooking is complete, hit Cancel. Allow the pressure to release naturally for 10 minutes, then quick release any remaining pressure.

8.   Unlock and remove lid.
9.   Spoon into serving bowls, sprinkle with cilantro or parsley, and serve.

**Per Serving (1½ cups)**
calories: 268 | fat: 10g | protein: 25g | carbs: 26g | sugars: 7g | fiber: 7g | sodium: 387mg

# BBQ Ribs and Broccoli Slaw

**Prep time: 10 minutes | Cook time: 50 minutes | Serves 6**

**BBQ Ribs:**
4 pounds (1.8 kg) baby back ribs
1 teaspoon freshly ground black pepper
½ cup plain 2 percent Greek yogurt
1 tablespoon olive oil
1 tablespoon fresh lemon juice
½ teaspoon fine sea salt
¼ teaspoon freshly ground black pepper
1 pound (454 g) broccoli florets (or florets from 2 large crowns), chopped
10 radishes, halved and thinly sliced
1 red bell pepper, seeded and cut lengthwise into narrow strips
1 large apple (such as Fuji, Jonagold, or Gala), thinly sliced
½ red onion, thinly sliced
**Finish:**
¾ cup low-sugar or unsweetened barbecue sauce

1 teaspoon fine sea salt
**Broccoli Slaw:**

1.   To make the ribs: Pat the ribs dry with paper towels, then cut the racks into six sections (three to five ribs per section, depending on how big the racks are). Season the ribs all over with the salt and pepper.
2.   Pour 1 cup water into the Instant Pot and place the wire metal steam rack into the pot. Place the ribs on top of the wire rack (it's fine to stack them up).
3.   Secure the lid and set the Pressure Release to Sealing. Select the Manual setting and set the cooking time for 20 minutes at high pressure. (The pot will take about 15 minutes to come up to pressure before the cooking program begins.)
4.   To make the broccoli slaw: While the ribs are cooking, in a small bowl, stir together the yogurt, oil, lemon juice, salt, and pepper, mixing well. In a large bowl, combine the broccoli, radishes, bell pepper, apple, and onion. Drizzle with the yogurt mixture and toss until evenly coated.
5.   When the ribs have about 10 minutes left in their cooking time, preheat the oven to 400ºF (205ºC). Line a sheet pan with aluminum foil.
6.   When the cooking program ends, perform a quick pressure release by moving the Pressure Release to Venting. Open the pot and, using tongs, transfer the ribs in a single layer to the prepared sheet pan. Brush the barbecue sauce onto both sides of the ribs, using 2 tablespoons of sauce per section of ribs. Bake, meaty-side up, for 15 to 20 minutes, until lightly browned.
7.   Serve the ribs warm, with the slaw on the side.

**Per Serving**
calories: 392 | fat: 15g | protein: 45g | carbs: 19g | sugars: 9g | fiber: 4g | sodium: 961mg

# "Smothered" Steak

**Prep time: 20 minutes | Cook time: 15 minutes | Serves 6**

1 tablespoon olive oil

⅓ cup flour

1½ pounds (680 g) chuck, or round, steak, cut into strips, trimmed of fat

1 large onion, sliced

1 (14½-ounce / 411-g) can stewed tomatoes

2 tablespoons soy sauce

beans

¼ teaspoon pepper

1 green pepper, sliced

1 (4-ounce / 113-g) can mushrooms, drained

1 (10-ounce / 283-g) package frozen French-style green

1. Press Sauté and add the oil to the Instant Pot.
2. Mix together the flour and pepper in a small bowl. Place the steak pieces into the mixture in the bowl and coat each of them well.
3. Lightly brown each of the steak pieces in the Instant Pot, about 2 minutes on each side. Press Cancel when done.
4. Add the remaining ingredients to the Instant Pot and mix together gently.
5. Secure the lid and make sure vent is set to sealing. Press Manual and set for 15 minutes.
6. When cook time is up, let the pressure release naturally for 15 minutes, then perform a quick release.

**Per Serving**

calories: 386 | fat: 24g | protein: 25g | carbs: 20g | sugars: 4g | fiber: 4g | sodium: 746mg

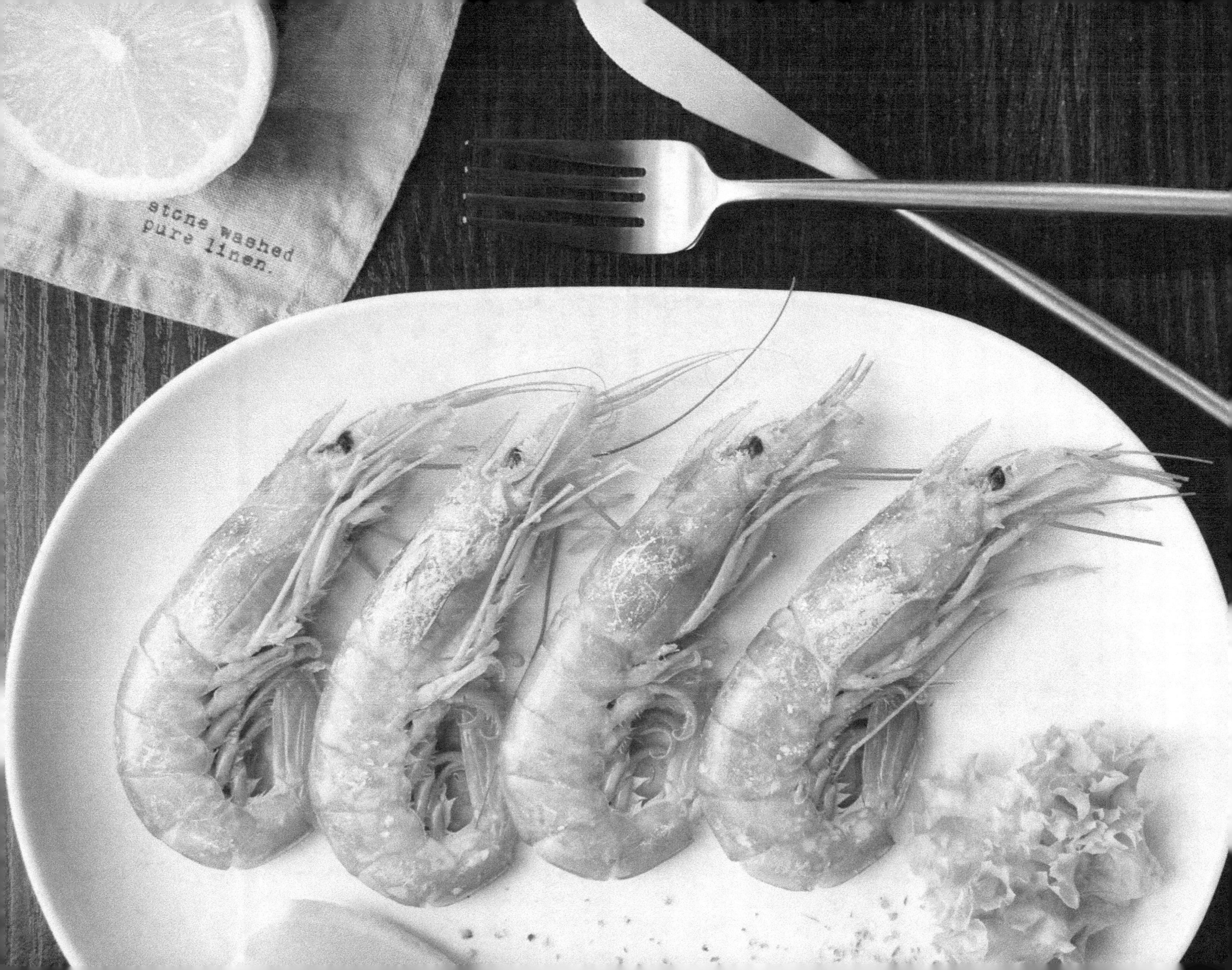

stone washed
pure linen.

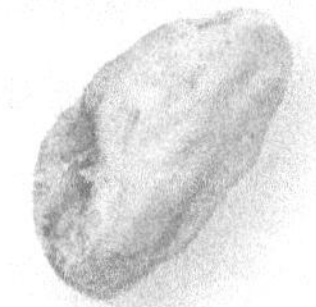


128   *Salade Niçoise with Oil-Packed Tuna*   103

129   *Shrimp Louie Salad with Thousand Island Dressing*   104

130   *Asian Cod with Brown Rice, Asparagus, and Mushrooms*   105

131   *Mediterranean Salmon with Whole-Wheat Couscous*   106

132   *Lemon Pepper Tilapia with Broccoli and Carrots*   107


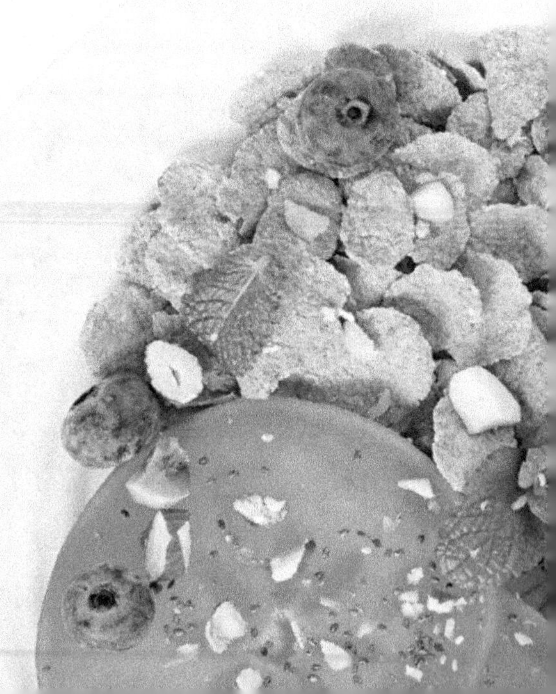

# Salade Niçoise with Oil-Packed Tuna

**Prep time: 5 minutes | Cook time: 20 minutes | Serves 4**

8 ounces (227 g) small red potatoes, quartered
8 ounces (227 g) green beans, trimmed
4 large eggs
French Vinaigrette:
2 tablespoons extra-virgin olive oil
2 tablespoons cold-pressed avocado oil
2 tablespoons white wine vinegar
1 tablespoon water
1 teaspoon Dijon mustard
½ teaspoon dried oregano
¼ teaspoon fine sea salt
1 tablespoon minced shallot

2 hearts romaine lettuce, leaves separated and torn into bite-size pieces
½ cup grape tomatoes, halved
¼ cup pitted Niçoise or Greek olives
1 (7-ounce / 198-g) can oil-packed tuna, drained and flaked
Freshly ground black pepper, to taste
1 tablespoon chopped fresh flat-leaf parsley

1. Pour 1 cup water into the Instant Pot and place a steamer basket into the pot. Add the potatoes, green beans, and eggs to the basket.
2. Secure the lid and set the Pressure Release to Sealing. Select the Steam setting and set the cooking time for 3 minutes at high pressure. (The pot will take about 15 minutes to come up to pressure before the cooking program begins.)
3. To make the vinaigrette: While the vegetables and eggs are steaming, in a small jar or other small container with a tight-fitting lid, combine the olive oil, avocado oil, vinegar, water, mustard, oregano, salt, and shallot and shake vigorously to emulsify. Set aside.
4. Prepare an ice bath.
5. When the cooking program ends, perform a quick release by moving the Pressure Release to Venting. Open the pot and, wearing heat-resistant mitts, lift out the steamer basket. Using tongs, transfer the eggs and green beans to the ice bath, leaving the potatoes in the steamer basket.
6. While the eggs and green beans are cooling, divide the lettuce, tomatoes, olives, and tuna among four shallow individual bowls. Drain the eggs and green beans. Peel and halve the eggs lengthwise, then arrange them on the salads along with the green beans and potatoes.
7. Spoon the vinaigrette over the salads and sprinkle with the pepper and parsley. Serve right away.

**Per Serving**
calories: 367 | fat: 23g | protein: 20g | carbs: 23g | sugars: 7g | fiber: 4g | sodium: 268mg

# Shrimp Louie Salad with Thousand Island Dressing

**Prep time: 5 minutes | Cook time: 20 minutes | Serves 4**

2 cups water

1 pound (454 g) medium shrimp, peeled and deveined

4 large eggs

**Thousand Island Dressing:**

¼ cup no-sugar-added ketchup

1 tablespoon fresh lemon juice

⅛ teaspoon cayenne pepper

2 green onions, white and green parts, sliced thinly

1½ teaspoons fine sea salt

¼ cup mayonnaise

1 teaspoon Worcestershire sauce

Freshly ground black pepper, to taste

2 hearts romaine lettuce or 1 head iceberg lettuce, shredded

1 English cucumber, sliced

1 cup cherry tomatoes, sliced

8 radishes, sliced

1 large avocado, pitted, peeled, and sliced

1.  Combine the water and salt in the Instant Pot and stir to dissolve the salt.
2.  Secure the lid and set the Pressure Release to Sealing. Select the Steam setting and set the cooking time for 0 (zero) minutes at low pressure. (The pot will take about 10 minutes to come up to pressure before the cooking program begins.)
3.  Meanwhile, prepare an ice bath.
4.  When the cooking program ends, perform a quick release by moving the Pressure Release to Venting. Open the pot and stir in the shrimp, using a wooden spoon to nudge them all down into the water. Cover the pot and leave the shrimp for 2 minutes on the Keep Warm setting. The shrimp will gently poach and cook through. Uncover the pot and, wearing heat-resistant mitts, lift out the inner pot and drain the shrimp in a colander. Transfer them to the ice bath to cool for 5 minutes, then drain them in the colander and set aside in the refrigerator.
5.  Rinse out the inner pot and return it to the housing. Pour in 1 cup water and place the wire metal steam rack into the pot. Place the eggs on top of the steam rack.
6.  Secure the lid and set the Pressure Release to Sealing. Press the Cancel button to reset the cooking program, then select the Manual setting and set the cooking time for 5 minutes at high pressure. (The pot will take about 5 minutes to come up to pressure before the cooking program begins.)
7.  While the eggs are cooking, prepare another ice bath.
8.  When the cooking program ends, let the pressure release naturally for 5 minutes, then move the Pressure Release to Venting to release any remaining steam. Using tongs, transfer the eggs to the ice bath and let cool for 5 minutes.
9.  To make the dressing: In a small bowl, stir together the ketchup, mayonnaise, lemon juice, Worcestershire sauce, cayenne, ¼ teaspoon black pepper, and green onions.
10. Arrange the lettuce, cucumber, radishes, tomatoes, and avocado on individual plates or in large, shallow individual bowls. Mound the cooked shrimp in the center of each salad. Peel the eggs, quarter them lengthwise, and place the quarters around the shrimp.
11. Spoon the dressing over the salads and top with additional black pepper. Serve right away.

**Per Serving**

calories: 407 | fat: 23g | protein: 35g | carbs: 16g | sugars: 10g | fiber: 6g | sodium: 1099mg

# Asian Cod with Brown Rice, Asparagus, and Mushrooms

**Prep time: 5 minutes | Cook time: 25 minutes | Serves 2**

¾ cup Minute brand brown rice

½ cup water

2 (5-ounce / 142-g) skinless cod fillets

1 tablespoon soy sauce or tamari

1 tablespoon fresh lemon juice

½ teaspoon peeled and grated fresh ginger

1 tablespoon extra-virgin olive oil or 1 tablespoon unsalted butter, cut into 8 pieces

2 green onions, white and green parts, thinly sliced

12 ounces (340 g) asparagus, trimmed

4 ounces (113 g) shiitake mushrooms, stems removed and sliced

⅛ teaspoon fine sea salt

⅛ teaspoon freshly ground black pepper

Lemon wedges, for serving

1. Pour 1 cup water into the Instant Pot. Have ready two-tier stackable stainless-steel containers.
2. In one of the containers, combine the rice and ½ cup water, then gently shake the container to spread the rice into an even layer, making sure all of the grains are submerged. Place the fish fillets on top of the rice. In a small bowl, stir together the soy sauce, lemon juice, and ginger. Pour the soy sauce mixture over the fillets. Drizzle 1 teaspoon olive oil on each fillet (or top with two pieces of the butter), and sprinkle the green onions on and around the fish.
3. In the second container, arrange the asparagus in the center in as even a layer as possible. Place the mushrooms on either side of the asparagus. Drizzle with the remaining 2 teaspoons olive oil (or put the remaining six pieces butter on top of the asparagus, spacing them evenly). Sprinkle the salt and pepper evenly over the vegetables.
4. Place the container with the rice and fish on the bottom and the vegetable container on top. Cover the top container with its lid and then latch the containers together. Grasping the handle, lower the containers into the Instant Pot.
5. Secure the lid and set the Pressure Release to Sealing. Select the Manual setting and set the cooking time for 15 minutes at high pressure. (The pot will take about 10 minutes to come up to pressure before the cooking program begins.)
6. When the cooking program ends, let the pressure release naturally for 5 minutes, then move the Pressure Release to Venting to release any remaining steam. Open the pot and, wearing heat-resistant mitts, lift out the stacked containers. Unlatch, unstack, and open the containers, taking care not to get burned by the steam.
7. Transfer the vegetables, rice, and fish to plates and serve right away, with the lemon wedges on the side.

**Per Serving**

calories: 344 | fat: 11g | protein: 27g | carbs: 46g | sugars: 6g | fiber: 7g | sodium: 637mg

# Mediterranean Salmon with Whole-Wheat Couscous

**Prep time: 5 minutes | Cook time: 30 minutes | Serves 4**

**Couscous:**
1 cup whole-wheat couscous
1 cup water
1 tablespoon extra-virgin olive oil
1 teaspoon dried basil
¼ teaspoon fine sea salt
1 pint cherry or grape tomatoes, halved
8 ounces (227 g) zucchini, halved lengthwise, then sliced crosswise ¼ inch thick
**Salmon:**
1 pound (454 g) skinless salmon fillet
2 teaspoons extra-virgin olive oil
1 tablespoon fresh lemon juice
1 garlic clove, minced
¼ teaspoon dried oregano
¼ teaspoon fine sea salt
¼ teaspoon freshly ground black pepper
1 tablespoon capers, drained
Lemon wedges, for serving

1. Pour 1 cup water into the Instant Pot. Have ready two-tier stackable stainless-steel containers.
2. To make the couscous: In one of the containers, stir together the couscous, water, oil, basil, and salt. Sprinkle the tomatoes and zucchini over the top.
3. To make the salmon: Place the salmon fillet in the second container. In a small bowl, whisk together the oil, lemon juice, garlic, oregano, salt, pepper, and capers. Spoon the oil mixture over the top of the salmon.
4. Place the container with the couscous and vegetables on the bottom and the salmon container on top. Cover the top container with its lid and then latch the containers together. Grasping the handle, lower the containers into the Instant Pot.
5. Secure the lid and set the Pressure Release to Sealing. Select the Manual setting and set the cooking time for 20 minutes at high pressure. (The pot will take about 10 minutes to come up to pressure before the cooking program begins.)
6. When the cooking program ends, let the pressure release naturally for 5 minutes, then move the Pressure Release to Venting to release any remaining steam. Open the pot and, wearing heat-resistant mitts, lift out the stacked containers. Unlatch, unstack, and open the containers, taking care not to get burned by the steam.
7. Using a fork, fluff the couscous and mix in the vegetables. Spoon the couscous onto plates, then use a spatula to cut the salmon into four pieces and place a piece on top of each couscous serving. Serve right away, with lemon wedges on the side.

## Per Serving
calories: 427 | fat: 18g | protein: 28g | carbs: 36g | sugars: 2g | fiber: 6g | sodium: 404mg

# Lemon Pepper Tilapia with Broccoli and Carrots

**Prep time: 15 minutes | Cook time: 15 minutes | Serves 4**

1 pound (454 g) tilapia fillets
1 teaspoon lemon pepper seasoning
¼ teaspoon fine sea salt
2 tablespoons extra-virgin olive oil
2 garlic cloves, minced
1 small yellow onion, sliced
½ cup low-sodium vegetable broth
2 tablespoons fresh lemon juice
1 pound (454 g) broccoli crowns, cut into bite-size florets
8 ounces (227 g) carrots, cut into ¼-inch thick rounds

1. Sprinkle the tilapia fillets all over with the lemon pepper seasoning and salt.
2. Select the Sauté setting on the Instant Pot and heat the oil and garlic for 2 minutes, until the garlic is bubbling but not browned. Add the onion and sauté for about 3 minutes more, until it begins to soften.
3. Pour in the broth and lemon juice, then use a wooden spoon to nudge any browned bits from the bottom of the pot. Using tongs, add the fish fillets to the pot in a single layer; it's fine if they overlap slightly. Place the broccoli and carrots on top.
4. Secure the lid and set the Pressure Release to Sealing. Press the Cancel button to reset the cooking program, then select the Manual setting and set the cooking time for 1 minute at low pressure. (The pot will take about 10 minutes to come up to pressure before the cooking program begins.)
5. When the cooking program ends, let the pressure release naturally for 10 minutes (don't open the pot before the 10 minutes are up, even if the float valve has gone down), then move the Pressure Release to Venting to release any remaining steam. Open the pot. Use a fish spatula to transfer the vegetables and fillets to plates. Serve right away.

**Per Serving**
calories: 243 | fat: 9g | protein: 28g | carbs: 15g | sugars: 4g | fiber: 5g | sodium: 348mg

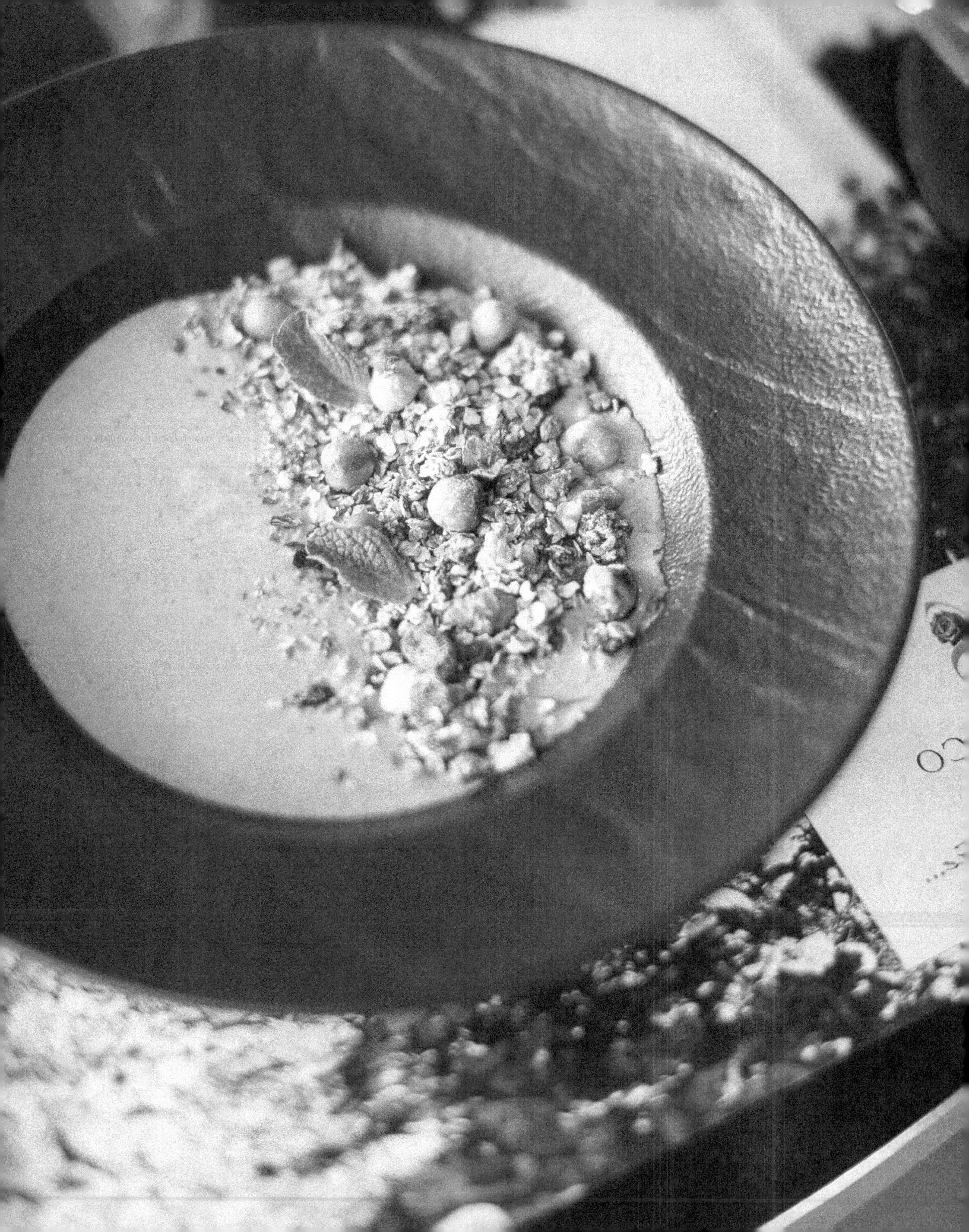

## Chapter 11 Desserts

133    **Crustless Key Lime Cheesecake**    110

134    **Chocolate Chocolate Chip Bundt Cake**    111

135    **Greek Yogurt Strawberry Pops**    112

136    **Fudgy Walnut Brownies**    112

137    **Almond Butter Blondies**    113

138    **New York Cheesecake**    114

# Crustless Key Lime Cheesecake

**Prep time: 15 minutes | Cook time: 35 minutes | Serves 8**

Nonstick cooking spray

16 ounces (454 g) light cream cheese (Neufchâtel), softened

⅔ cup granulated erythritol sweetener

¼ cup unsweetened Key lime juice

½ teaspoon vanilla extract

¼ cup plain Greek yogurt

1 teaspoon grated lime zest

2 large eggs

Whipped cream, for garnish (optional)


1. Spray a 7-inch springform pan with nonstick cooking spray. Line the bottom and partway up the sides of the pan with foil.
2. Put the cream cheese in a large bowl. Use an electric mixer to whip the cream cheese until smooth, about 2 minutes. Add the erythritol, lime juice, vanilla, yogurt, and zest, and blend until smooth. Stop the mixer and scrape down the sides of the bowl with a rubber spatula. With the mixer on low speed, add the eggs, one at a time, blending until just mixed. (Don't overbeat the eggs.)
3. Pour the mixture into the prepared pan. Drape a paper towel over the top of the pan, not touching the cream cheese mixture, and tightly wrap the top of the pan in foil. (Your goal here is to keep out as much moisture as possible.)
4. Pour 1 cup of water into the electric pressure cooker.
5. Place the foil-covered pan onto the wire rack and carefully lower it into the pot.
6. Close and lock the lid of the pressure cooker. Set the valve to sealing.
7. Cook on high pressure for 35 minutes.
8. When the cooking is complete, hit Cancel. Allow the pressure to release naturally for 20 minutes, then quick release any remaining pressure.
9. Once the pin drops, unlock and remove the lid.
10. Using the handles of the wire rack, carefully transfer the pan to a cooling rack. Cool to room temperature, then refrigerate for at least 3 hours.
11. When ready to serve, run a thin rubber spatula around the rim of the cheesecake to loosen it, then remove the ring.
12. Slice into wedges and serve with whipped cream (if using).


**Per Serving (1 slice)**

calories: 157 | fat: 12g | protein: 8g | carbs: 4g | sugars: 1g | fiber: 0g | sodium: 196mg

# Chocolate Chocolate Chip Bundt Cake

**Prep time: 10 minutes | Cook time: 50 minutes | Serves 8**

1¼ cups Bob's Red Mill paleo flour

⅔ cup Lakanto Monkfruit Sweetener Golden

⅓ cup natural cocoa powder

1½ teaspoons baking powder

½ teaspoon fine sea salt

3 large eggs

½ cup plain 2 percent Greek yogurt

¼ cup vegan shortening or unsalted butter, melted and cooled

1 teaspoon pure vanilla extract          ½ cup stevia-sweetened chocolate chips

1. Pour 1 cup water into the Instant Pot. Grease a 7-inch Bundt pan with shortening or unsalted butter, then lightly coat the inside of the pan with flour, tapping out any excess.

2. In a large bowl, whisk together the flour, sweetener, cocoa powder, baking powder, and salt. Add the eggs, Greek yogurt, shortening, and vanilla and whisk just until incorporated. Using a spoon or rubber spatula, fold in the chocolate chips.

3. Transfer the batter to the prepared pan and, using the spoon or spatula, spread it in an even layer. Cover the pan tightly with aluminum foil. Place the pan on a long-handled silicone steam rack, then, holding the handles of the steam rack, lower it into the Instant Pot. (If you don't have the long-handled rack, use the wire metal steam rack and a homemade sling)

4. Secure the lid and set the Pressure Release to Sealing. Select the Manual setting and set the cooking time for 40 minutes at high pressure. (The pot will take about 10 minutes to come up to pressure before the cooking program begins.)

5. When the cooking program ends, let the pressure release naturally for 10 minutes, then move the Pressure Release to Venting to release any remaining steam. Open the pot and, wearing heat-resistant mitts, grasp the handles of the steam rack, lift it out of the pot, and set it on a cooling rack. Uncover the pan, taking care not to get burned by the steam or to drip condensation onto the cake. Let the cake cool for 10 minutes, then invert it onto the cooling rack and lift off the pan. Let cool for about 50 minutes, to room temperature.

6. Transfer the cake to a serving plate. Cut into eight slices and serve.

**Per Serving**

calories: 209 | fat: 15g | protein: 7g | carbs: 33g | sugars: 11g | fiber: 22g | sodium: 202mg

# Greek Yogurt Strawberry Pops



2 ripe bananas, peeled, cut into ½-inch pieces, and frozen
½ cup plain 2 percent Greek yogurt
1 cup chopped fresh strawberries

1. In a food processor, combine the bananas and yogurt and process at high speed for 2 minutes, until mostly smooth (it's okay if a few small chunks remain). Scrape down the sides of the bowl, add the strawberries, and process for 1 minute, until smooth.
2. Divide the mixture evenly among six ice-pop molds. Tap each mold on a countertop a few times to get rid of any air pockets, then place an ice-pop stick into each mold and transfer the molds to the freezer. Freeze for at least 4 hours, or until frozen solid.
3. To unmold each ice pop, run it under cold running water for 5 seconds, taking care not to get water inside the mold, then remove the ice pop from the mold. Eat the ice pops right away or store in a ziplock plastic freezer bag in the freezer for up to 2 months.

**Per Serving**
calories: 57 | fat: 1g | protein: 3g | carbs: 12g | sugars: 6g | fiber: 2g | sodium: 8mg

# Fudgy Walnut Brownies



¾ cup walnut halves and pieces
4 large eggs
1½ teaspoons vanilla extract
¼ teaspoon fine sea salt
¾ cup natural cocoa powder

½ cup unsalted butter, melted and cooled
1½ teaspoons instant coffee crystals
1 cup Lakanto Monkfruit Sweetener Golden
¾ cup almond flour
¾ cup stevia-sweetened chocolate chips

1. In a dry small skillet over medium heat, toast the walnuts, stirring often, for about 5 minutes, until golden. Transfer the walnuts to a bowl to cool.
2. Pour 1 cup water into the Instant Pot. Line the base of a 7 by 3-inch round cake pan with a circle of parchment paper. Butter the sides of the pan and the parchment or coat with nonstick cooking spray.
3. Pour the butter into a medium bowl. One at a time, whisk in the eggs, then whisk in the coffee crystals, vanilla, sweetener, and salt. Finally, whisk in the flour and cocoa powder just until combined. Using a rubber spatula, fold in the chocolate chips and walnuts.
4. Transfer the batter to the prepared pan and, using the spatula, spread it in an even layer. Cover the pan tightly with aluminum foil. Place the pan on a long-handled silicone steam rack, then, holding the handles of the steam rack, lower it into the Instant Pot.
5. Secure the lid and set the Pressure Release to Sealing. Select the Manual setting and set the cooking time for 45 minutes at high pressure. (The pot will take about 10 minutes to come up to pressure before the cooking program begins.)
6. When the cooking program ends, let the pressure release naturally for 10 minutes, then move the Pressure Release to Venting to release any remaining steam. Open the pot and, wearing heat-resistant mitts, grasp

the handles of the steam rack and lift it out of the pot. Uncover the pan, taking care not to get burned by the steam or to drip condensation onto the brownies. Let the brownies cool in the pan on a cooling rack for about 2 hours, to room temperature.

7.  Run a butter knife around the edge of the pan to make sure the brownies are not sticking to the pan sides. Invert the brownies onto the rack, lift off the pan, and peel off the parchment paper. Invert the brownies onto a serving plate and cut into twelve wedges. The brownies will keep, stored in an airtight container in the refrigerator for up to 5 days, or in the freezer for up to 4 months.

**Per Serving**
calories: 199 | fat: 19g | protein: 5g | carbs: 26g | sugars: 10g | fiber: 20g | sodium: 56mg

## Almond Butter Blondies

**Prep time: 10 minutes | Cook time: 20 minutes | Serves 8**

½ cup creamy natural almond butter, at room temperature
4 large eggs
¾ cup Lakanto Monkfruit Sweetener Golden
1 teaspoon pure vanilla extract
½ teaspoon fine sea salt
1¼ cups almond flour
¾ cup stevia-sweetened chocolate chips

1.  Pour 1 cup water into the Instant Pot. Line the base of a 7 by 3-inch round cake pan with a circle of parchment paper. Butter the sides of the pan and the parchment or coat with nonstick cooking spray.
2.  Put the almond butter into a medium bowl. One at a time, whisk the eggs into the almond butter, then whisk in the sweetener, vanilla, and salt. Stir in the flour just until it is fully incorporated, followed by the chocolate chips.
3.  Transfer the batter to the prepared pan and, using a rubber spatula, spread it in an even layer. Cover the pan tightly with aluminum foil. Place the pan on a long-handled silicone steam rack, then, holding the handles of the steam rack, lower it into the Instant Pot.
4.  Secure the lid and set the Pressure Release to Sealing. Select the Manual setting and set the cooking time for 40 minutes at high pressure. (The pot will take about 10 minutes to come up to pressure before the cooking program begins.)
5.  When the cooking program ends, let the pressure release naturally for 10 minutes, then move the Pressure Release to Venting to release any remaining steam. Open the pot and, wearing heat-resistant mitts, grasp the handles of the steam rack and lift it out of the pot. Uncover the pan, taking care not to get burned by the steam or to drip condensation onto the blondies. Let the blondies cool in the pan on a cooling rack for about 5 minutes.
6.  Run a butter knife around the edge of pan to make sure the blondies are not sticking to the pan sides. Invert the blondies onto the rack, lift off the pan, and peel off the parchment paper. Let cool for 15 minutes, then invert the blondies onto a serving plate and cut into eight wedges. The blondies will keep, stored in an airtight container in the refrigerator for up to 5 days, or in the freezer for up to 4 months.

**Per Serving**
calories: 211 | fat: 17g | protein: 8g | carbs: 20g | sugars: 10g | fiber: 17g | sodium: 186mg

# New York Cheesecake

**Prep time: 15 minutes | Cook time: 45 minutes | Serves 8**

## Crust:

4 graham cracker sheets (gluten-free, if desired)          ¼ cup pecans or pecan pieces
1 tablespoon unsalted butter, melted and cooled

## Filling:

1 (8-ounce / 227-g) package cream cheese, at room temperature
¾ cup plain 2 percent Greek yogurt, at room temperature
½ cup Lakanto Monkfruit Sweetener Golden or Classic
1 teaspoon pure vanilla extract          3 large eggs, at room temperature

1 cup fresh raspberries or sliced fresh strawberries

1.  Line the base of a 7 by 3-inch round removable-bottom cake pan or springform pan with an 8-inch round of parchment paper. If using a springform pan, secure its collar, clamping down the parchment paper and securing the collar onto the base. Lightly butter the sides of the pan or coat with nonstick cooking spray.
2.  To make the crust: In a food processor, process the graham crackers to fine crumbs. Add the pecans and melted butter. Using 1-second pulses, process until the mixture resembles damp sand.
3.  Transfer the crumb mixture to the prepared pan and press it firmly into an even layer onto the bottom and about ½ inch up the sides of the pan. Wipe out the food processor.
4.  To make the filling: In the food processor, combine the cream cheese, yogurt, sweetener, and vanilla. Process using about five 1-second pulses, just until smooth, stopping to scrape down the sides of the bowl as needed. One at a time, add the eggs, processing with two 1-second pulses after each addition. Do not overprocess the filling, or the batter may overflow the pan and/or you will end up with an overly fluffy cheesecake. Using a rubber spatula, gently stir in any large streaks of egg yolk. It's fine if a few small streaks remain.
5.  Pour the filling into the prepared crust. Tap the pan firmly against the countertop a few times to remove any air bubbles in the filling. Cover the pan tightly with aluminum foil. Place the pan on a long-handled silicone steam rack. (If you don't have the long-handled rack, use the wire metal steam rack and a homemade sling)
6.  Pour 1½ cups water into the Instant Pot. Holding the handles of the steam rack, lower the pan into the pot.
7.  Secure the lid and set the Pressure Release to Sealing. Select the Manual setting and set the cooking time for 32 minutes at high pressure. (The pot will take about 10 minutes to come up to pressure before the cooking program begins.)
8.  When the cooking program ends, let the pressure release naturally for 20 minutes, then move the Pressure Release to Venting to release any remaining steam. Open the pot and, wearing heat-resistant mitts, grasp the handles of the steam rack, lift it out of the pot, and set the pan on a cooling rack. Remove the foil, taking care not to get burned by the steam or to drip condensation onto the cheesecake. Use a paper towel to dab up any moisture that may have settled on the surface. The cake will be puffed up and may look a bit uneven when it comes out of the pot, but it will settle and set up as it cools. Let the cheesecake cool on the rack for about 2 hours, then cover and refrigerate for at least 12 hours or up to 24 hours.
9.  Run a butter knife around the edge of the pan to make sure the crust is not sticking to the pan sides. If using a removable-bottom cake pan, set the pan atop a widemouthed jar or can and gently pull downward on the pan ring. If using a springform pan, unclasp the collar and lift if off. Use the parchment border to tug the cheesecake off the pan bottom and onto a serving plate.
10.  Cut the cheesecake into eight slices and serve with the berries on the side.

**Per Serving (cheesecake only)**
calories: 219 | fat: 17g | protein: 7g | carbs: 21g | sugars: 11g | fiber: 13g | sodium: 141mg

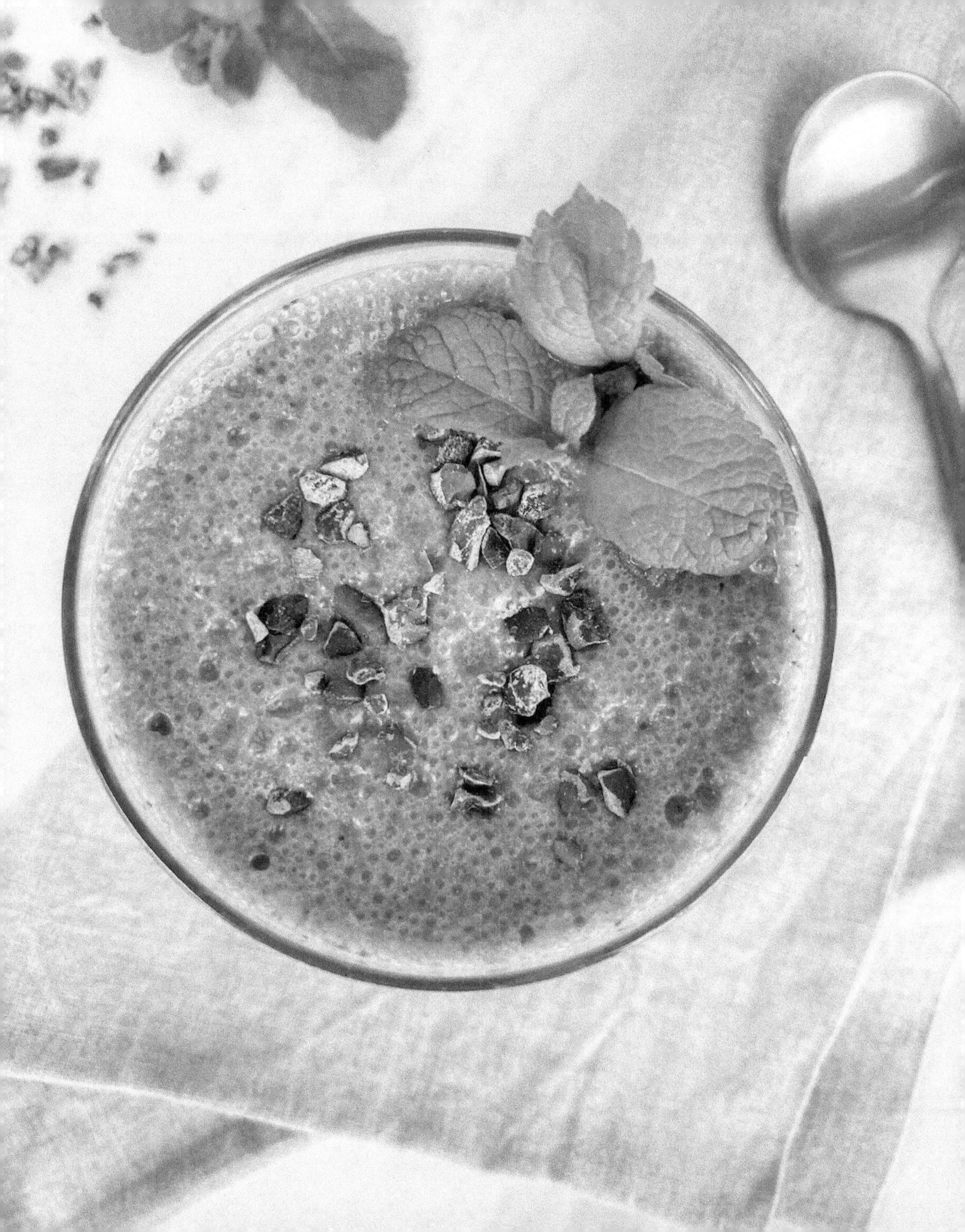

# Chapter 12 Staples

139    Vegetable Broth    117

140    Cashew Ranch Dip    117

141    Chicken Bone Broth    118

142    Spiced Tomato Ketchup    118

143    Cornbread    119

144    Roasted Tomatillo Salsa    120

145    Low-Sodium Salsa    120

146    Garam Masala    120

147    5-Minute Pesto    121

148    Italian Turkey Sausage Meatballs    121

149    Low-Sodium Roasted Beef Bone Broth    122

150    Toasted Nuts    122



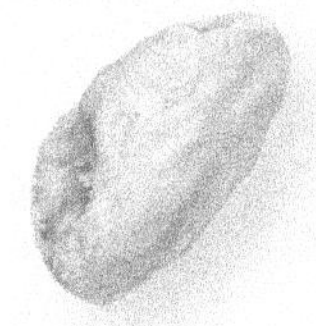

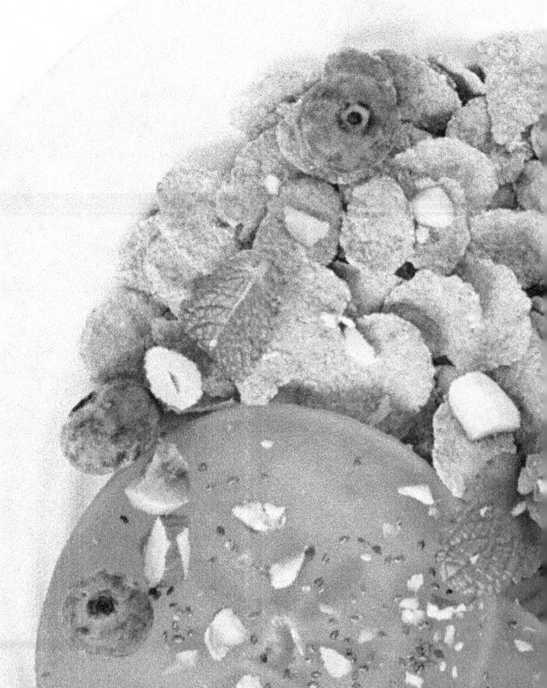

# Vegetable Broth



**Prep time: 10 minutes | Cook time: 15 minutes | Makes 8 cups**

2 or 3 (4-inch) rosemary sprigs

2 or 3 (4-inch) thyme sprigs

2 or 3 (4-inch) parsley sprigs

1 large onion (unpeeled), root end trimmed, quartered

2 large carrots (unpeeled), washed, ends trimmed, and each cut into 4 pieces

2 celery stalks (including leaves), ends trimmed and each cut into 4 pieces

4 garlic cloves, peeled and left whole

2 bay leaves

½ teaspoon peppercorns

1.  Using kitchen twine, tie together the rosemary, thyme, and parsley. (If you don't have twine, don't worry about it. Tying the herbs together just makes it easier to discard them later.)
2.  In the electric pressure cooker, combine the onion, carrots, celery, garlic, bay leaves, and peppercorns. Drop the herb bundle on top, then pour in 6 cups of water.
3.  Close and lock the lid of the pressure cooker. Set the valve to sealing.
4.  Cook on high pressure for 15 minutes.
5.  When the cooking is complete, hit Cancel. Allow the pressure to release naturally for 15 minutes, then quick release any remaining pressure.
6.  Once the pin drops, unlock and remove the lid.
7.  Cool the broth to room temperature, then strain it through a fine-mesh strainer lined with cheesecloth. Discard the solids.
8.  Transfer to storage containers and refrigerate for 3 to 4 days or freeze for up to 1 year.

**Per Serving (1 cup)**

calories: 12 | fat: 0g | protein: 0g | carbs: 3g | sugars: 1g | fiber: 1g | sodium: 17mg

# Cashew Ranch Dip

**Prep time: 1 minute | Cook time: 1 hour | Makes 2 cups**

1 cup raw whole cashews, soaked in water to cover for 1 to 2 hours and then drained

½ cup water

2 tablespoons fresh lemon juice

1 teaspoon nutritional yeast

1 teaspoon garlic powder

½ teaspoon fine sea salt

½ teaspoon freshly ground black pepper

1 tablespoon chopped fresh chives

1 tablespoon chopped fresh dill

1 tablespoon chopped fresh flat-leaf parsley

1.  In a blender, combine the cashews, water, lemon juice, nutritional yeast, garlic powder, salt, and pepper. Blend on high speed for about 1 minute, until very smooth, stopping to scrape down the sides if needed.
2.  Transfer the dip to a bowl and stir in the chives, dill, and parsley. Cover and refrigerate for at least 1 hour before serving. The dip will keep in the refrigerator for up to 5 days. If it becomes too thick, stir in a splash of water.

**Per Serving (2 tablespoons)**

calories: 44 | fat: 3g | protein: 1g | carbs: 3g | sugars: 0g | fiber: 0g | sodium: 171mg

# Chicken Bone Broth

**Prep time: 11 minutes | Cook time: 2 hours | Makes 8 cups**

2 or 3 (4-inch) rosemary sprigs

2 or 3 (4-inch) thyme sprigs

2 or 3 (4-inch) parsley sprigs

Bones from a 3- to 4-pound (1.4- to 1.8-kg) chicken

1 large onion (unpeeled), root end trimmed, quartered

2 large carrots (unpeeled), washed, ends trimmed, and each cut into 4 pieces

2 celery stalks (including leaves), ends trimmed and each cut into 4 pieces

2 bay leaves

⅛ teaspoon black peppercorns

1 teaspoon kosher salt (optional)

1 tablespoon apple cider vinegar

1. Using kitchen twine, tie together the rosemary, thyme, and parsley. (If you don't have any twine, don't worry about it. Tying the herbs together just makes it easier to discard them later.)
2. In the electric pressure cooker, combine the bones, onion, carrots, celery, bay leaves, peppercorns, and salt (if using). Drop the herb bundle on top, then add the vinegar and 8 cups of water.
3. Close and lock the lid of the pressure cooker. Set the valve to sealing.
4. Cook on high pressure for 2 hours.
5. When the cooking is complete, hit Cancel. Allow the pressure to release naturally for 20 minutes, then quick release any remaining pressure.
6. Once the pin drops, unlock and remove the lid.
7. Cool the broth to room temperature, then strain it through a fine-mesh strainer lined with cheesecloth. Discard the solids.
8. Transfer to storage containers and refrigerate for 3 to 4 days, or freeze for up to 1 year.

**Per Serving (1 cup)**
calories: 40 | fat: 1g | protein: 6g | carbs: 3g | sugars: 0g | fiber: 1g | sodium: 20mg

# Spiced Tomato Ketchup

**Prep time: 10 minutes | Cook time: 15 minutes | Makes 4 cups**

1 (28-ounce / 794-g) carton or can crushed tomatoes

1 (6-ounce / 170-g) can tomato paste

½ cup finely chopped onion

½ cup cider vinegar

¼ cup pure maple syrup

½ teaspoon dry mustard (such as Colman's)

¼ teaspoon ground allspice

¼ teaspoon ground cinnamon

¼ teaspoon ground mace

¼ teaspoon ground ginger

¼ teaspoon ground cloves

¼ teaspoon red pepper flakes (optional)

¼ teaspoon kosher salt

Freshly ground black pepper, to taste

1. In the electric pressure cooker, combine the tomatoes, tomato paste, onion, vinegar, maple syrup, mustard, allspice, cinnamon, mace, ginger, cloves, red pepper flakes (if using), salt, and pepper. Stir well.
2. Close and lock the lid of the pressure cooker. Set the valve to sealing.
3. Cook on high pressure for 15 minutes.
4. When the cooking is complete, hit Cancel. Allow the pressure to release naturally for 10 minutes, then quick release any remaining pressure.
5. Once the pin drops, unlock and remove the lid.

6. Use an immersion blender right in the pot to get the ketchup to a nice, thick consistency. If it looks watery at all, hit Sauté and let the ketchup simmer until it is the correct thickness. It should fall off of a spoon while slightly resisting.

7. Let the ketchup cool to room temperature, then store it, covered, in the refrigerator for up to 2 months.

**Per Serving (2 tablespoons)**
calories: 21 | fat: 0g | protein: 1g | carbs: 5g | sugars: 3g | fiber: 1g | sodium: 90mg

# Cornbread

**Prep time: 10 minutes | Cook time: 45 minutes | Serves 8**

**1 cup almond flour**
**½ cup cornmeal**
**¼ cup coconut flour**
**2 teaspoons baking powder**
**1 teaspoon fine sea salt**
**2 large eggs**
**1 cup unsweetened almond milk**
**4 tablespoons vegan shortening or unsalted butter, melted and cooled**

1. Pour 1 cup water into the Instant Pot. Grease the bottom and sides of a 7-inch round cake pan with shortening or butter.

2. In a medium bowl, whisk together the almond flour, cornmeal, coconut flour, baking powder, and salt. In another medium bowl, whisk together the eggs and almond milk until no streaks of yolk remain.

3. Add the egg mixture and shortening to the almond flour mixture and whisk just until the dry ingredients are evenly and fully moistened. The coconut flour absorbs moisture quickly, so the batter will thicken as it sits.

4. Transfer the batter to the prepared pan and, using a rubber spatula, spread it in an even layer. Cover the pan tightly with aluminum foil. Place the pan on a long-handled silicone steam rack, then, holding the handles of the steam rack, lower it into the Instant Pot. (If you don't have the long-handled rack, use the wire metal steam rack and a homemade sling)

5. Secure the lid and set the Pressure Release to Sealing. Select the Manual setting and set the cooking time for 35 minutes at high pressure. (The pot will take about 10 minutes to come up to pressure before the cooking program begins.)

6. When the cooking program ends, let the pressure release naturally for 10 minutes, then move the Pressure Release to Venting to release any remaining steam. Open the pot and, wearing heat-resistant mitts, grasp the handles of the steam rack, lift it out of the pot, and set it on a cooling rack. Uncover the pan, taking care not to get burned by the steam or to drip condensation onto the bread. Let the bread cool for 5 minutes, then run a butter knife around the edge of the pan to loosen the bread from the pan sides. Invert the bread onto the cooling rack, lift off the pan, and invert the bread onto a serving plate.

7. Cut the bread into eight wedges and serve warm.

**Per Serving**
calories: 230 | fat: 17g | protein: 6g | carbs: 14g | sugars: 1g | fiber: 3g | sodium: 309mg

# Roasted Tomatillo Salsa

**Prep time: 5 minutes | Cook time: 1 hour | Makes 1 cup**

1 pound (454 g) tomatillos (about 6 large), papery husks removed, rinsed
½ large onion, quartered
1 tablespoon extra-virgin olive oil
1 cup (loosely packed) fresh cilantro leaves
3 serrano chiles, halved lengthwise, seeded
1 teaspoon kosher salt

1.  Preheat the oven to 375ºF (190ºC).
2.  In an 8-inch square baking dish, combine the tomatillos, onion, chiles, oil, and salt. Roast for 1 hour or until the vegetables are very soft. Remove from the oven and let cool slightly.
3.  Transfer everything from the baking dish to a food processor, and add the cilantro. Purée until almost smooth. Pour the salsa into a glass jar and store, covered, in the refrigerator for up to 1 week.

**Per Serving (2 tablespoons)**
calories: 33 | fat: 2g | protein: 1g | carbs: 4g | sugars: 2g | fiber: 1g | sodium: 187mg

# Low-Sodium Salsa

**Prep time: 10 minutes | Cook time: 10 minutes | Makes 1 cup**

8 ounces (227 g) cocktail tomatoes, quartered
2 scallions, white and light green parts only, chopped
1 jalapeño chile, seeded and chopped
1 tablespoon freshly squeezed lime juice
2 tablespoons chopped fresh cilantro

1.  In a food processor, combine the tomatoes, scallions, jalapeño, cilantro, and lime juice. Pulse until the salsa is the consistency you like. If you don't have a food processor, finely chop the tomatoes, scallions, and jalapeño, then mix with the cilantro and lime juice.
2.  Store, covered, in the refrigerator for up to 3 days.

**Per Serving (2 tablespoons)**
calories: 7 | fat: 0g | protein: 0g | carbs: 2g | sugars: 1g | fiber: 1g | sodium: 2mg

# Garam Masala

**Prep time: 5 minutes | Cook time: 0 minutes | Makes ⅓ cup**

2 tablespoons ground cumin
1 tablespoon freshly ground black pepper
1 tablespoon ground cardamom
1 tablespoon ground coriander
2 teaspoons ground cinnamon
1 teaspoon ground nutmeg
1 teaspoon ground cloves
⅛ teaspoon cayenne pepper (optional)

1. In an old spice jar or small bowl, combine the cumin, black pepper, cardamom, coriander, cinnamon, nutmeg, cloves, and cayenne (if using). Mix well and store, covered and in a cool, dry location, for up to 6 months.

**Per Serving (1½ tablespoons)**
calories: 32 | fat: 1g | protein: 1g | carbs: 6g | sugars: 0g | fiber: 3g | sodium: 7mg

## 5-Minute Pesto

**Prep time: 5 minutes | Cook time: 0 minutes | Makes 1 cup**

3 garlic cloves, peeled
½ cup freshly grated Parmesan cheese
½ cup extra-virgin olive oil
Freshly ground black pepper, to taste

2 cups packed fresh basil leaves
⅓ cup pine nuts
Kosher salt, to taste

1. With the motor running, drop the garlic cloves through the feed tube of a food processor fitted with the steel blade. Stop the motor, then add the basil, Parmesan, and pine nuts. Pulse a few times until the pine nuts are finely minced.
2. With the motor running, add the olive oil in a steady stream and process until the pesto is completely puréed. Season with salt and pepper.
3. Store, covered, in the refrigerator for up to 2 weeks.

**Per Serving (1 tablespoon)**
calories: 94 | fat: 10g | protein: 2g | carbs: 1g | sugars: 0g | fiber: 0g | sodium: 71mg

## Italian Turkey Sausage Meatballs

**Prep time: 15 minutes | Cook time: 25 minutes | Makes about 24 meatballs**

1 pound (454 g) ground chicken
8 ounces (227 g) Italian turkey sausage (hot or sweet), casings removed
⅔ cup Italian-style bread crumbs
3 tablespoons chopped fresh parsley
3 tablespoons nonfat milk
1 teaspoon kosher salt

2 teaspoons minced garlic
½ cup freshly grated Parmesan cheese
1 large egg, lightly beaten
½ teaspoon freshly ground black pepper

1. Preheat the oven to 350ºF (180ºC).
2. In a large bowl, combine the chicken, sausage, bread crumbs, garlic, parsley, Parmesan, milk, egg, salt, and pepper. Mix gently but thoroughly. (I like to use my hands.)
3. Line a sheet pan with parchment paper. Pinch off about 1 tablespoon of the meat mixture and roll it into a ball. A 1¼-inch cookie scoop makes the job easy. Place the meatball on the sheet pan and repeat with the remaining meat. You should end up with about 24 meatballs.
4. If you plan to eat the meatballs right away, bake them for 30 minutes or until they are lightly browned and cooked through. If you plan to freeze the meatballs, bake them for 20 minutes, then let them cool before freezing.

**Per Serving (4 meatballs)**
calories: 269 | fat: 13g | protein: 25g | carbs: 12g | sugars: 3g | fiber: 1g | sodium: 877mg

# Low-Sodium Roasted Beef Bone Broth

**Prep time: 15 minutes | Cook time: 3 hours 15 minutes | Makes 8 cups**

2 pounds (907 g) beef soup bones (such as knucklebones, shanks, or oxtails)
2 celery stalks, cut into 3-inch lengths
1 parsnip or 2 large carrots, halved lengthwise, then cut crosswise into 3-inch lengths
1 yellow onion, cut into wedges
½ teaspoon black peppercorns
1 tablespoon tomato paste
8 cups water
1 teaspoon fine sea salt
2 bay leaves
1 tablespoon raw apple cider vinegar

1.  Preheat the oven to 400ºF (205ºC). Line a large sheet pan with aluminum foil.
2.  Arrange the beef bones in a single layer on the prepared pan. Roast for about 45 minutes, until browned.
3.  Using tongs, transfer the roasted bones to the Instant Pot. Add the celery, parsnip, onion, salt, peppercorns, bay leaves, tomato paste, and vinegar. Slowly pour in the water to prevent splashing. Make sure the pot is no more than two-thirds full.
4.  Secure the lid and set the Pressure Release to Sealing. Select the Soup or Manual setting and set the cooking time for 120 minutes at high pressure. (The pot will take about 30 minutes to come up to pressure before the cooking program begins.)
5.  When the cooking program ends, let the pressure release naturally; this will take about 45 minutes.
6.  Place a fine-mesh strainer over a large heatproof bowl or pitcher. For a clearer broth, line the strainer with a double layer of cheesecloth.
7.  Open the pot and, using tongs, remove the bones. Wearing heat-resistant mitts, lift out the inner pot and pour the broth through the strainer. Discard the contents of the strainer. You can pick the meat off the bones if you like, but it will have given up most of its flavor to the broth. Pour the broth into a fat separator to remove the fat, then let the broth cool to room temperature. Alternatively, let the broth cool to room temperature, then chill in the refrigerator until the fat solidifies on top and scoop off the fat from the surface with a large spoon. (To speed up the cooling process, prepare an ice bath and set the bowl in the ice bath for about 15 minutes.)
8.  The broth can be used right away, or stored in an airtight container in the refrigerator for up to 5 days or in the freezer for up to 6 months.

**Per Serving (1 cup)**
calories: 30 | fat: 0g | protein: 6g | carbs: 1g | sugars: 1g | fiber: 0g | sodium: 313mg

# Toasted Nuts

**Prep time: 1 minute | Cook time: 8 minutes | Makes ½ cup**

½ cup nuts

1.  Heat a dry nonstick pan over medium-high heat.
2.  Place the nuts in the pan and toss or stir frequently for 2 to 5 minutes, until they are toasted and fragrant.
3.  Remove from the heat and let cool.

**Per Serving (1 tablespoon)**
calories: 40 | fat: 3g | protein: 1g | carbs: 2g | sugars: 0g | fiber: 1g | sodium: 0mg

# Appendix 1: Measurement Conversion Chart

## VOLUME EQUIVALENTS(DRY)

| US STANDARD | METRIC (APPROXIMATE) |
|---|---|
| 1/8 teaspoon | 0.5 mL |
| 1/4 teaspoon | 1 mL |
| 1/2 teaspoon | 2 mL |
| 3/4 teaspoon | 4 mL |
| 1 teaspoon | 5 mL |
| 1 tablespoon | 15 mL |
| 1/4 cup | 59 mL |
| 1/2 cup | 118 mL |
| 3/4 cup | 177 mL |
| 1 cup | 235 mL |
| 2 cups | 475 mL |
| 3 cups | 700 mL |
| 4 cups | 1 L |

## WEIGHT EQUIVALENTS

| US STANDARD | METRIC (APPROXIMATE) |
|---|---|
| 1 ounce | 28 g |
| 2 ounces | 57 g |
| 5 ounces | 142 g |
| 10 ounces | 284 g |
| 15 ounces | 425 g |
| 16 ounces (1 pound) | 455 g |
| 1.5 pounds | 680 g |
| 2 pounds | 907 g |

## VOLUME EQUIVALENTS(LIQUID)

| US STANDARD | US STANDARD (OUNCES) | METRIC (APPROXIMATE) |
|---|---|---|
| 2 tablespoons | 1 fl.oz. | 30 mL |
| 1/4 cup | 2 fl.oz. | 60 mL |
| 1/2 cup | 4 fl.oz. | 120 mL |
| 1 cup | 8 fl.oz. | 240 mL |
| 1 1/2 cup | 12 fl.oz. | 355 mL |
| 2 cups or 1 pint | 16 fl.oz. | 475 mL |
| 4 cups or 1 quart | 32 fl.oz. | 1 L |
| 1 gallon | 128 fl.oz. | 4 L |

## TEMPERATURES EQUIVALENTS

| FAHRENHEIT(F) | CELSIUS(C) (APPROXIMATE) |
|---|---|
| 225 °F | 107 °C |
| 250 °F | 120 °C |
| 275 °F | 135 °C |
| 300 °F | 150 °C |
| 325 °F | 160 °C |
| 350 °F | 180 °C |
| 375 °F | 190 °C |
| 400 °F | 205 °C |
| 425 °F | 220 °C |
| 450 °F | 235 °C |
| 475 °F | 245 °C |
| 500 °F | 260 °C |

## Dried Beans, Legumes and Lentils

| Dried Beans and Legume | Dry (Minutes) | Soaked (Minutes) |
|---|---|---|
| Soy beans | 25 – 30 | 20 – 25 |
| Scarlet runner | 20 – 25 | 10 – 15 |
| Pinto beans | 25 – 30 | 20 – 25 |
| Peas | 15 – 20 | 10 – 15 |
| Navy beans | 25 – 30 | 20 – 25 |
| Lima beans | 20 – 25 | 10 – 15 |
| Lentils, split, yellow (moong dal) | 15 – 18 | N/A |
| Lentils, split, red | 15 – 18 | N/A |
| Lentils, mini, green (brown) | 15 – 20 | N/A |
| Lentils, French green | 15 – 20 | N/A |
| Kidney white beans | 35 – 40 | 20 – 25 |
| Kidney red beans | 25 – 30 | 20 – 25 |
| Great Northern beans | 25 – 30 | 20 – 25 |
| Pigeon peas | 20 – 25 | 15 – 20 |
| Chickpeas (garbanzo bean chickpeas) | 35 – 40 | 20 – 25 |
| Cannellini beans | 35 – 40 | 20 – 25 |
| Black-eyed peas | 20 – 25 | 10 – 15 |
| Black beans | 20 – 25 | 10 – 15 |

## Fish and Seafood

| Fish and Seafood | Fresh (minutes) | Frozen (minutes) |
|---|---|---|
| Shrimp or Prawn | 1 to 2 | 2 to 3 |
| Seafood soup or stock | 6 to 7 | 7 to 9 |
| Mussels | 2 to 3 | 4 to 6 |
| Lobster | 3 to 4 | 4 to 6 |
| Fish, whole (snapper, trout, etc.) | 5 to 6 | 7 to 10 |
| Fish steak | 3 to 4 | 4 to 6 |
| Fish fillet, | 2 to 3 | 3 to 4 |
| Crab | 3 to 4 | 5 to 6 |

## Fruits

| Fruits | Fresh (in Minutes) | Dried (in Minutes) |
|---|---|---|
| Raisins | N/A | 4 to 5 |
| Prunes | 2 to 3 | 4 to 5 |
| Pears, whole | 3 to 4 | 4 to 6 |
| Pears, slices or halves | 2 to 3 | 4 to 5 |
| Peaches | 2 to 3 | 4 to 5 |
| Apricots, whole or halves | 2 to 3 | 3 to 4 |
| Apples, whole | 3 to 4 | 4 to 6 |
| Apples, in slices or pieces | 2 to 3 | 3 to 4 |

## Meat

| Meat and Cuts | Cooking Time (minutes) | Meat and Cuts | Cooking Time (minutes) |
|---|---|---|---|
| Veal, roast | 35 to 45 | Duck, with bones, cut up | 10 to 12 |
| Veal, chops | 5 to 8 | Cornish Hen, whole | 10 to 15 |
| Turkey, drumsticks (leg) | 15 to 20 | Chicken, whole | 20 to 25 |
| Turkey, breast, whole, with bones | 25 to 30 | Chicken, legs, drumsticks, or thighs | 10 to 15 |
| Turkey, breast, boneless | 15 to 20 | Chicken, with bones, cut up | 10 to 15 |
| Quail, whole | 8 to 10 | Chicken, breasts | 8 to 10 |
| Pork, ribs | 20 to 25 | Beef, stew | 15 to 20 |
| Pork, loin roast | 55 to 60 | Beef, shanks | 25 to 30 |
| Pork, butt roast | 45 to 50 | Beef, ribs | 25 to 30 |
| Pheasant | 20 to 25 | Beef, steak, pot roast, round, rump, brisket or blade, small chunks, chuck, | 25 to 30 |
| Lamb, stew meat | 10 to 15 | | |
| Lamb, leg | 35 to 45 | Beef, pot roast, steak, rump, round, chuck, blade or brisket, large | 35 to 40 |
| Lamb, cubes, | 10 t0 15 | | |
| Ham slice | 9 to 12 | Beef, ox-tail | 40 to 50 |
| Ham picnic shoulder | 25 to 30 | Beef, meatball | 10 to 15 |
| Duck, whole | 25 to 30 | Beef, dressed | 20 to 25 |

| Vegetable | Fresh (minutes) | Frozen (minutes) | Vegetable | Fresh (minutes) | Frozen (minutes) |
|---|---|---|---|---|---|
| Zucchini, slices or chunks | 2 to 3 | 3 to 4 | Mixed vegetables | 2 to 3 | 3 to 4 |
| Yam, whole, small | 10 to 12 | 12 to 14 | Leeks | 2 to 4 | 3 to 5 |
| Yam, whole, large | 12 to 15 | 15 to 19 | Greens (collards, beet greens, spinach, kale, turnip greens, swiss chard) chopped | 3 to 6 | 4 to 7 |
| Yam, in cubes | 7 to 9 | 9 to 11 | | | |
| Turnip, chunks | 2 to 4 | 4 to 6 | Green beans, whole | 2 to 3 | 3 to 4 |
| Tomatoes, whole | 3 to 5 | 5 to 7 | Escarole, chopped | 1 to 2 | 2 to 3 |
| Tomatoes, in quarters | 2 to 3 | 4 to 5 | Endive | 1 to 2 | 2 to 3 |
| Sweet potato, whole, small | 10 to 12 | 12 to 14 | Eggplant, chunks or slices | 2 to 3 | 3 to 4 |
| Sweet potato, whole, large | 12 to 15 | 15 to 19 | Corn, on the cob | 3 to 4 | 4 to 5 |
| Sweet potato, in cubes | 7 to 9 | 9 to 11 | Corn, kernels | 1 to 2 | 2 to 3 |
| Sweet pepper, slices or chunks | 1 to 3 | 2 to 4 | Collard | 4 to 5 | 5 to 6 |
| Squash, butternut, slices or chunks | 8 to 10 | 10 to 12 | Celery, chunks | 2 to 3 | 3 to 4 |
| Squash, acorn, slices or chunks | 6 to 7 | 8 to 9 | Cauliflower flowerets | 2 to 3 | 3 to 4 |
| Spinach | 1 to 2 | 3 to 4 | Carrots, whole or chunked | 2 to 3 | 3 to 4 |
| Rutabaga, slices | 3 to 5 | 4 to 6 | Carrots, sliced or shredded | 1 to 2 | 2 to 3 |
| Rutabaga, chunks | 4 to 6 | 6 to 8 | Cabbage, red, purple or green, wedges | 3 to 4 | 4 to 5 |
| Pumpkin, small slices or chunks | 4 to 5 | 6 to 7 | Cabbage, red, purple or green, shredded | 2 to 3 | 3 to 4 |
| Pumpkin, large slices or chunks | 8 to 10 | 10 to 14 | Brussel sprouts, whole | 3 to 4 | 4 to 5 |
| Potatoes, whole, large | 12 to 15 | 15 to 19 | Broccoli, stalks | 3 to 4 | 4 to 5 |
| Potatoes, whole, baby | 10 to 12 | 12 to 14 | Broccoli, flowerets | 2 to 3 | 3 to 4 |
| Potatoes, in cubes | 7 to 9 | 9 to 11 | Beets, small roots, whole | 11 to 13 | 13 to 15 |
| Peas, in the pod | 1 to 2 | 2 to 3 | Beets, large roots, whole | 20 to 25 | 25 to 30 |
| Peas, green | 1 to 2 | 2 to 3 | Beans, green/yellow or wax, whole, trim ends and strings | 1 to 2 | 2 to 3 |
| Parsnips, sliced | 1 to 2 | 2 to 3 | | | |
| Parsnips, chunks | 2 to 4 | 4 to 6 | Asparagus, whole or cut | 1 to 2 | 2 to 3 |
| Onions, sliced | 2 to 3 | 3 to 4 | Artichoke, whole, trimmed without leaves | 9 to 11 | 11 to 13 |
| Okra | 2 to 3 | 3 to 4 | Artichoke, hearts | 4 to 5 | 5 to 6 |

## Rice and Grains

| Rice & Grain | Water Quantity (Grain: Water ratios) | Cooking Time (in Minutes) | Rice & Grain | Water Quantity (Grain: Water ratios) | Cooking Time (in Minutes) |
|---|---|---|---|---|---|
| Wheat berries | 1:3 | 25 to 30 | Oats, steel-cut | 1:1 | 10 |
| Spelt berries | 1:3 | 15 to 20 | Oats, quick cooking | 1:1 | 6 |
| Sorghum | 1:3 | 20 to 25 | Millet | 1:1 | 10 to 12 |
| Rice, wild | 1:3 | 25 to 30 | Kamut, whole | 1:3 | 10 to 12 |
| Rice, white | 1:1.5 | 8 | Couscous | 1:2 | 5 to 8 |
| Rice, Jasmine | 1:1 | 4 to 10 | Corn, dried, half | 1:3 | 25 to 30 |
| Rice, Brown | 1:1.3 | 22 to 28 | Congee, thin | 1:6 ~ 1:7 | 15 to 20 |
| Rice, Basmati | 1:1.5 | 4 to 8 | Congee, thick | 1:4 ~ 1:5 | 15 to 20 |
| Quinoa, quick cooking | 1:2 | 8 | Barley, pot | 1:3 ~ 1:4 | 25 to 30 |
| Porridge, thin | 1:6 ~ 1:7 | 15 to 20 | Barley, pearl | 1:4 | 25 to 30 |

# Appendix 3: The Dirty Dozen and Clean Fifteen

The Environmental Working Group (EWG) is a nonprofit, nonpartisan organization dedicated to protecting human health and the environment Its mission is to empower people to live healthier lives in a healthier environment. This organization publishes an annual list of the twelve kinds of produce, in sequence, that have the highest amount of pesticide residue-the Dirty Dozen-as well as a list of the fifteen kinds ofproduce that have the least amount of pesticide residue-the Clean Fifteen.

## THE DIRTY DOZEN

- The 2016 Dirty Dozen includes the following produce. These are considered among the year's most important produce to buy organic:

| | |
|---|---|
| Strawberries | Spinach |
| Apples | Tomatoes |
| Nectarines | Bell peppers |
| Peaches | Cherry tomatoes |
| Celery | Cucumbers |
| Grapes | Kale/collard greens |
| Cherries | Hot peppers |

- *The Dirty Dozen list contains two additional itemskale/collard greens and hot peppers-because they tend to contain trace levels of highly hazardous pesticides.*

## THE CLEAN FIFTEEN

- The least critical to buy organically are the Clean Fifteen list. The following are on the 2016 list:

| | |
|---|---|
| Avocados | Papayas |
| Corn | Kiw |
| Pineapples | Eggplant |
| Cabbage | Honeydew |
| Sweet peas | Grapefruit |
| Onions | Cantaloupe |
| Asparagus | Cauliflower |
| Mangos | |

- *Some of the sweet corn sold in the United States are made from genetically engineered (GE) seedstock. Buy organic varieties of these crops to avoid GE produce.*